Ultimate Guide to Outpatient Care

Edited by Gaffar Sarwar Zaman

Published in London, United Kingdom

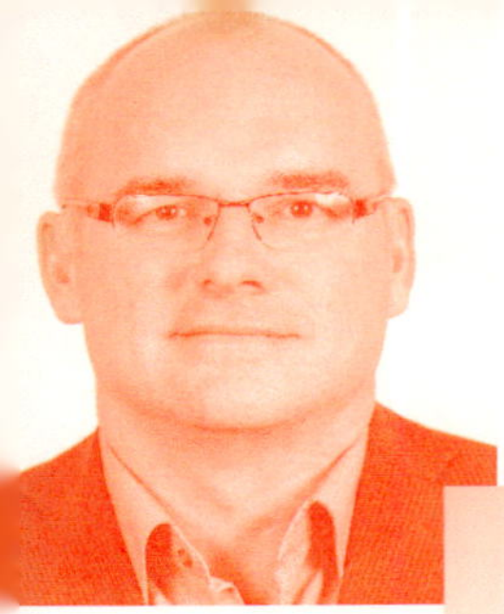
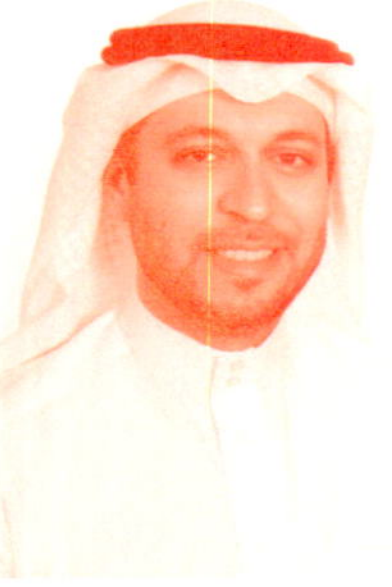
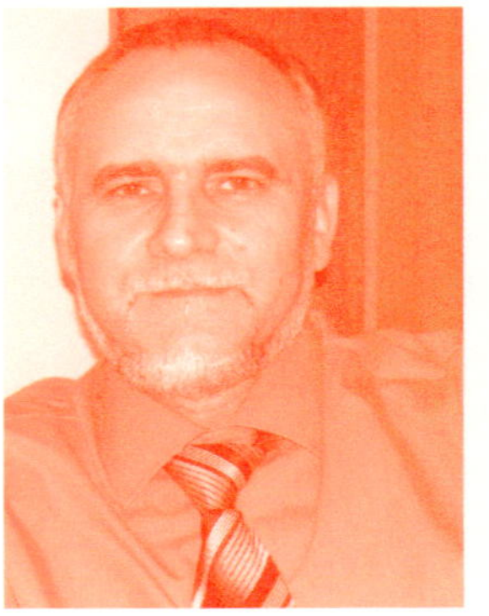
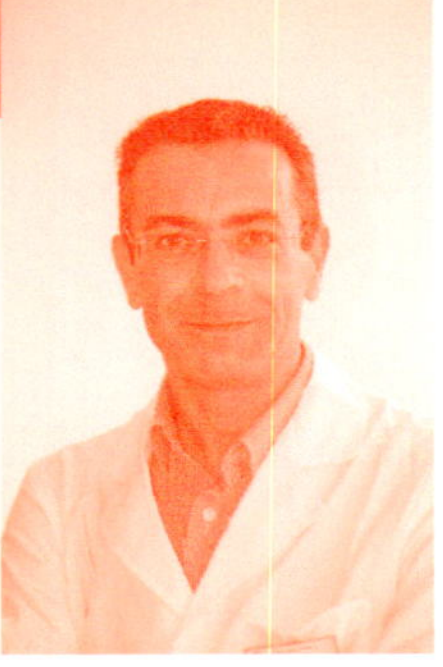
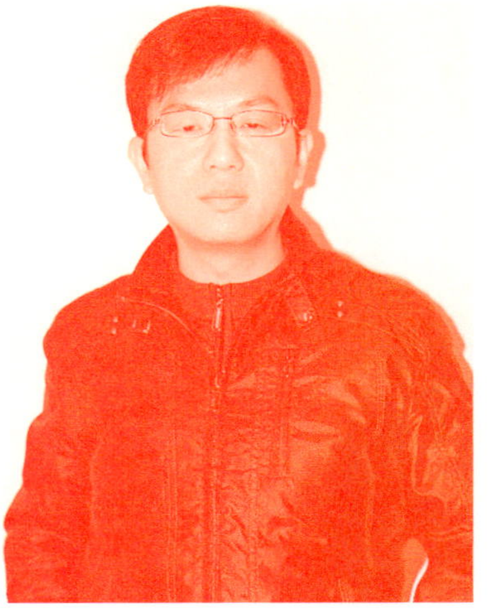
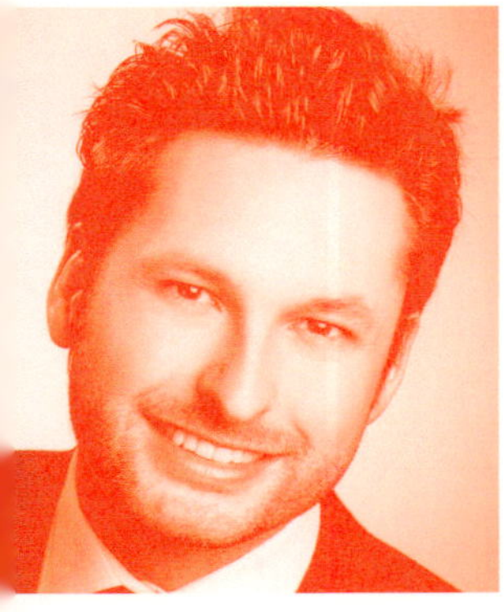
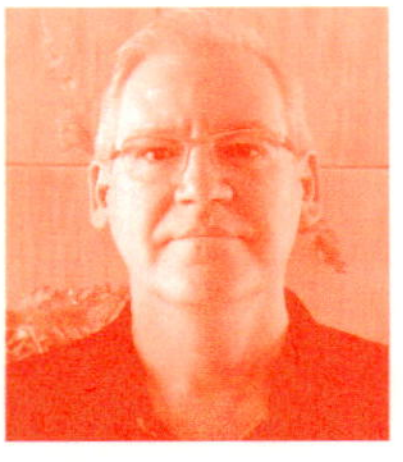

IntechOpen

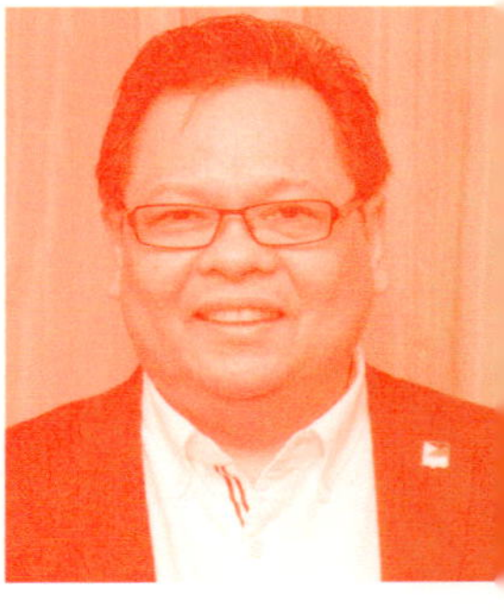
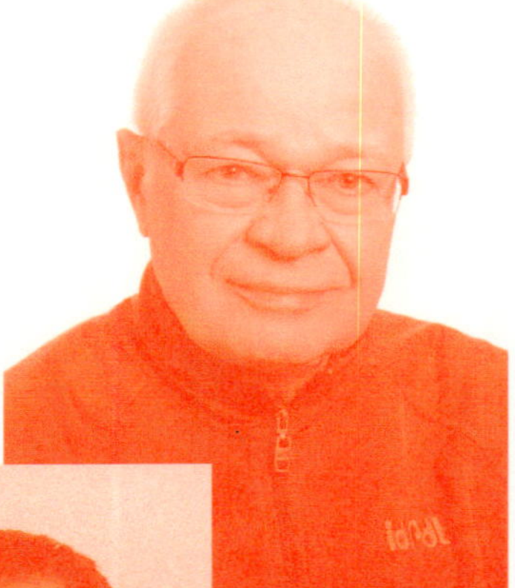
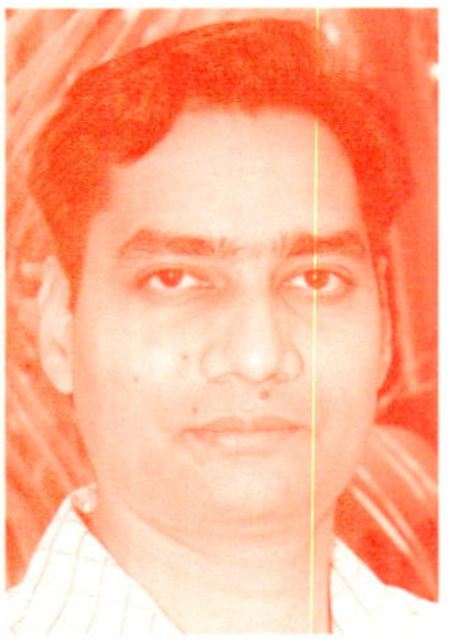
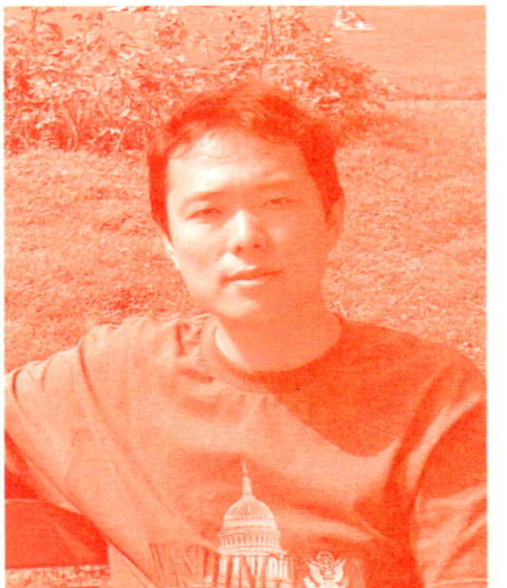
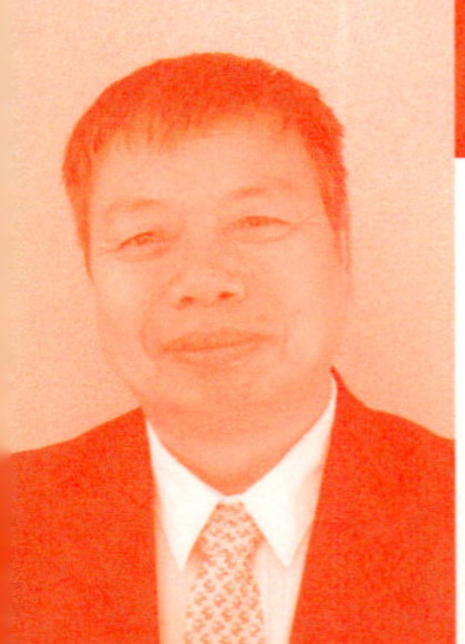
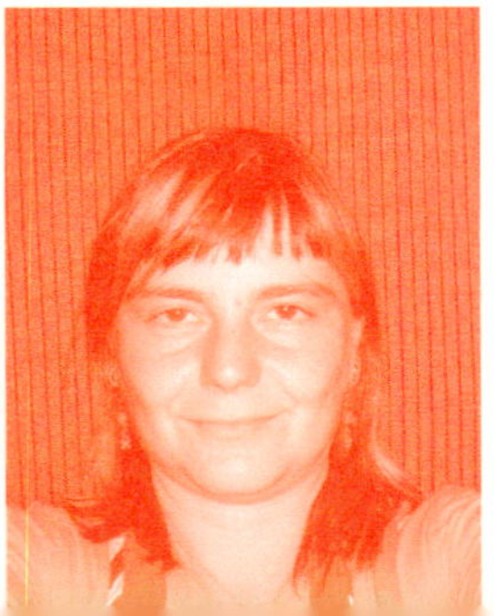

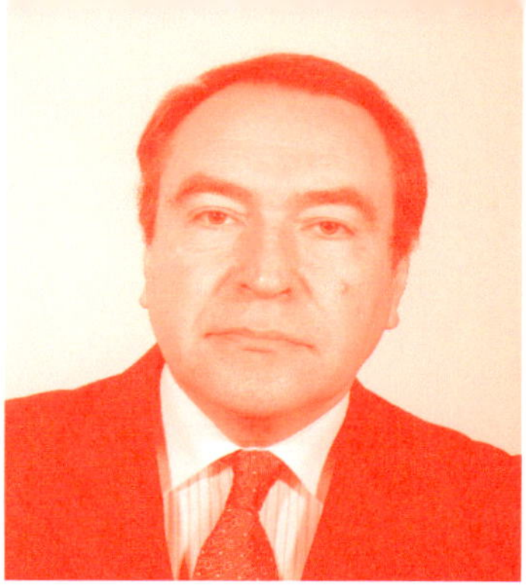
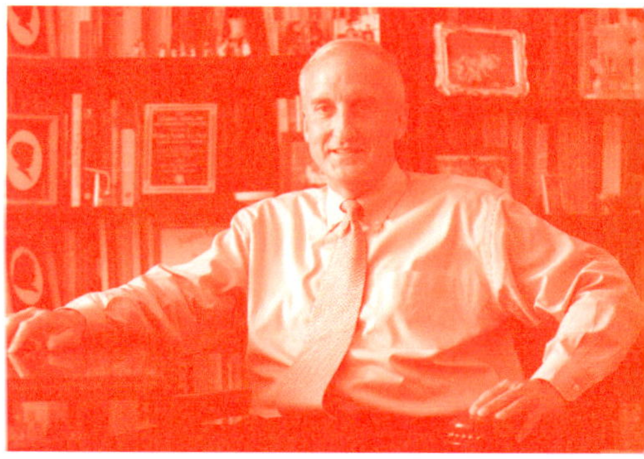
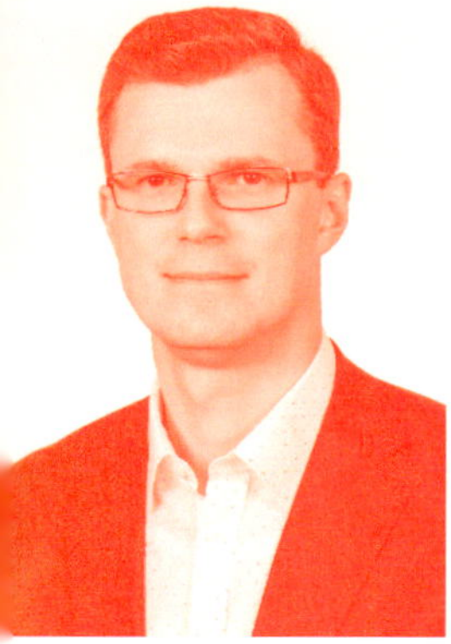
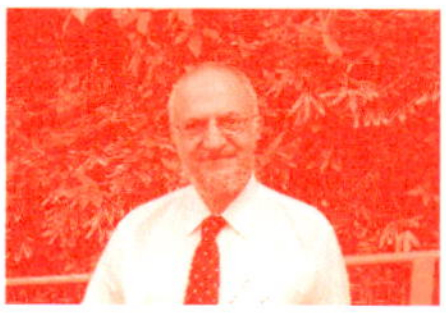
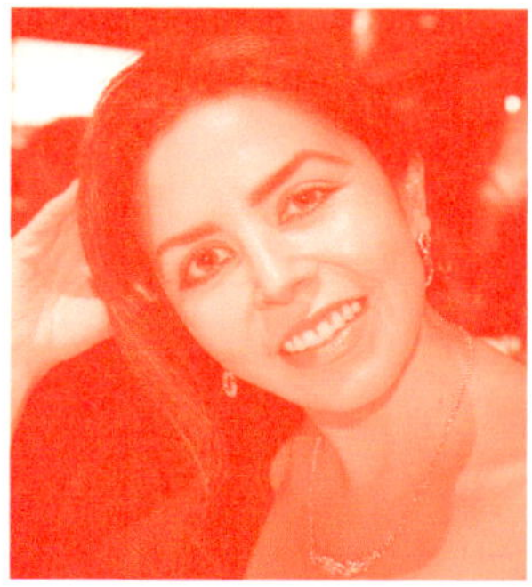

Supporting open minds since 2005

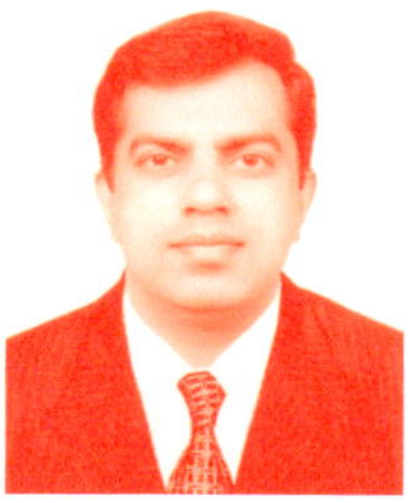
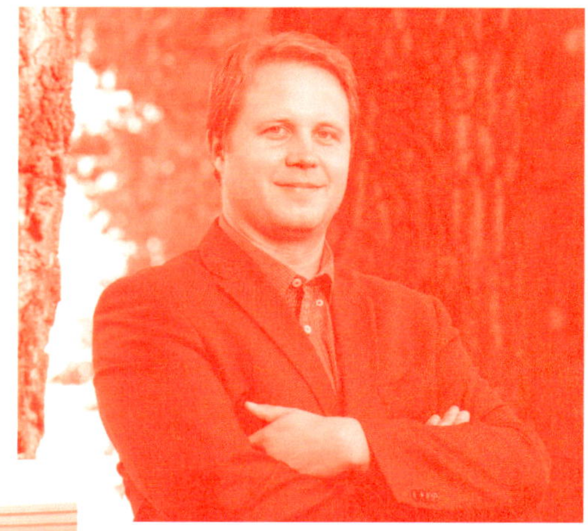
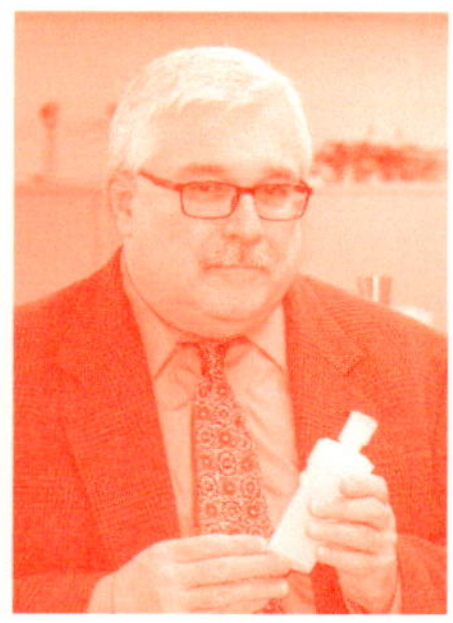
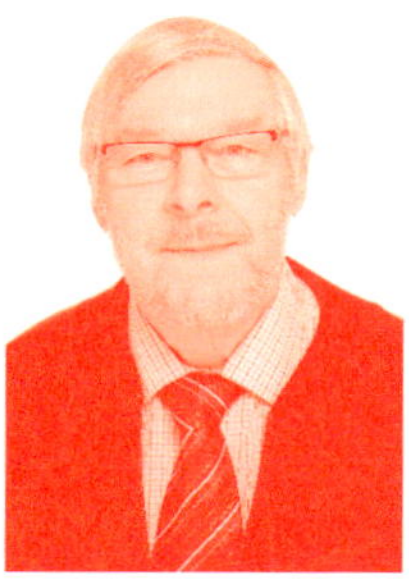
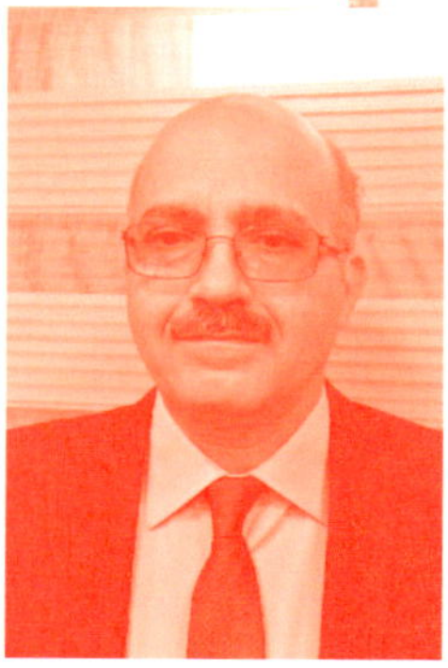
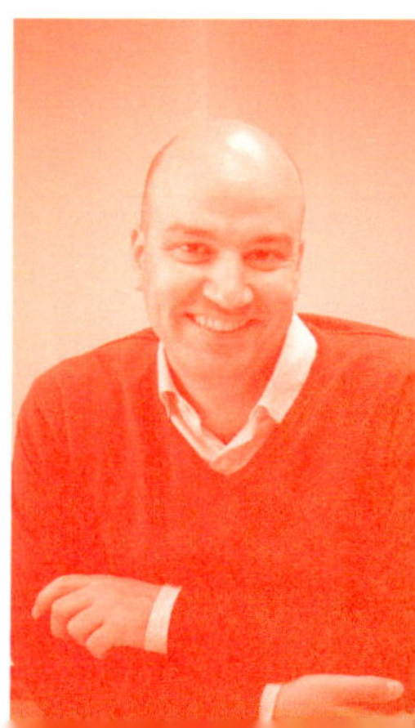
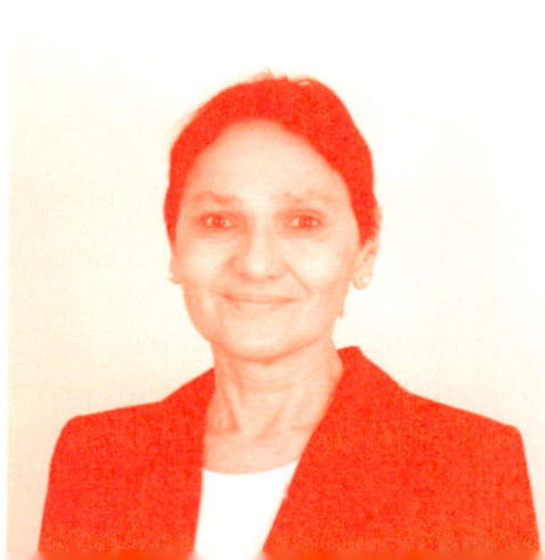

Ultimate Guide to Outpatient Care
http://dx.doi.org/10.5772/intechopen.87619
Edited by Gaffar Sarwar Zaman

Contributors
Ayesha Ajmi, Dilar Costa, Filipa Aguiar, Inés Llamas-Ramos, Rocío Llamas-Ramos, Jonathan Comyn De Rothewelle, Oleg Anatolievich Shtegman, Marina Mihailovna Petrova, Abimbola O. Asojo, Hoa Vo, Suyeon Bae, Chelsea Hetherington, Sarah Cronin, Judy Myers, Satyendra K. Tiwary, Andrea Divizia, Giuseppe S. Sica, Handan Eren

First published in London, United Kingdom, 2022 by IntechOpen
IntechOpen is the global imprint of INTECHOPEN LIMITED, registered in England and Wales, registration number: 11086078, 5 Princes Gate Court, London, SW7 2QJ, United Kingdom
Printed in Croatia

British Library Cataloguing-in-Publication Data
A catalogue record for this book is available from the British Library

Additional hard and PDF copies can be obtained from orders@intechopen.com

Ultimate Guide to Outpatient Care
Edited by Gaffar Sarwar Zaman
p. cm.
Print ISBN 978-1-83968-762-4
Online ISBN 978-1-83968-763-1
eBook (PDF) ISBN 978-1-83968-764-8

For EU product safety concerns:
IN TECH d.o.o., Prolaz Marije Krucifikse Kozulić 3, 51000 Rijeka, Croatia, info@intechopen.com or visit our website at intechopen.com.

Meet the editor

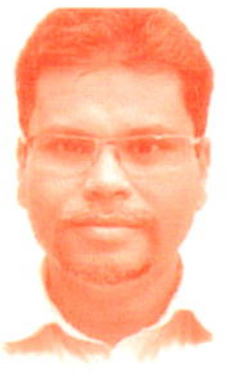

Dr. Zaman obtained an MD in Biochemistry from Assam Medical College & Hospital, Srimanta Sankaradeva University of Health Sciences (formerly under Dibrugarh University), India. He completed a Fellowship in Diabetes (FID) at Royal Liverpool Academy, United Kingdom, and a Fellowship in Applied Nutrition (FIAN) at Medvarsity, Apollo Hospitals, India. Dr. Zaman obtained a Post Graduate Diploma in Clinical Research (PGDCR) from Symbiosis University, India. He has almost fifteen years of experience as an Associate Professor Professor at King Khalid Government University, Saudi Arabia, and Rajiv Gandhi University of Health Sciences, India. He has expertise in quality development and curriculum design and is trained in e-learning methods. He has more than fifty research publications to his credit in both national and international journals. He has also edited/co-edited books and authored many book chapters.

Contents

Preface

Patients who do not require hospitalization or overnight stay in the hospital can be treated via outpatient care; these patients are known as outpatients. Patients who attend appointments at a hospital or clinic for any check-up or aftercare following treatment are also considered outpatients. The popularity of outpatient care has increased because of technological advancements such as minimally invasive surgery. Ear, nose, and throat (ENT), heart, kidney, and orthopedic surgeries can be performed at outpatient facilities because of these new techniques. Technology and patient consumerism are two of the top factors contributing to the growth of outpatient facilities such as ambulatory surgery centers (ASCs), primary care clinics, and urgent care centers, according to Definitive Healthcare's 2019 outpatient trends report. Hospital-based outpatient services can be broadly classified into five main types: clinical, surgical, emergency, home health, and women's health. Other types of outpatient services include school health, office health, outpatient mental health, and others that are newly emerging. Recently, telemedicine-based follow-up has proven to be feasible and safe for the evaluation of early postoperative complications. Patients reported high levels of satisfaction with the experience. As such, telemedicine-based follow-up could become standard practice with the development of mobile applications. One of the most facilitative aspects of outpatient care is that it can be accomplished in non-medical institution-based settings, such as schools, prisons, offices, and more. Outpatient care is likely to become even more popular with the advancement of technology to support it.

This work would not have been possible without the support of IntechOpen. I am especially indebted to Author Service Manager Mr. Josip Knapić, who has been supportive of this project and who worked actively to provide me with all facilities. I am grateful to all of those with whom I have had the pleasure to work during this project. Each of the chapter authors provided me with extensive professional help and obliged me on this scientific venture wherever possible. Nobody has been more important to me in the pursuit of this project than the members of my family. I would like to thank my late parents, Taufiquz Zaman and Jaiba Zaman, whose love and guidance are with me in whatever I pursue. Most importantly, I wish to thank my loving and supportive wife, Mrs. Jarin Tanwir Hussain, who is my ultimate role model, and my two wonderful children, Naushad Muntasir Zaman and Umar Sarwar Zaman, who provided me with unending inspiration during the preparation and publication of this book.

Dr. Gaffar Sarwar Zaman, MBBS, MD
Fellowship in Diabetology,
Fellowship in Applied Nutrition,
PGDCR,
Associate Professor,
Department of Clinical Laboratory Sciences,
Government College of Applied Medical Sciences,
King Khalid University,
Abha, Kingdom of Saudi Arabia

Chapter 1

Needling Therapies in the Outpatient Care: Adverse Effects

Inés Llamas-Ramos and Rocío Llamas-Ramos

Abstract

The invasive techniques have been used for many years. There is a lot of literature on the advances that have been made, as well as the adverse effects or possible complications that have occurred during the performance of these treatments. Acupuncture and injections (saline, anesthetics, corticosteroids or botulinum toxin) have reported several cases of complications. Dry needling is also beginning to have several publications of this type. The objective of this chapter is to summarize the articles published in relation to adverse effects of needling therapies to promote a good practice and knowledge. Original articles in form of randomized controlled trials, case reports and reviews relating adverse effects and possible complications due to invasive/needling techniques: acupuncture, injections and dry needling have been included. 102 articles met the inclusion criteria between January 2000 and January 2020. The first limitation found in the literature was the huge variety of cases, therapists and incidents to generalize. As a conclusion we can stated the importance of a good knowledge of the anatomy and its variants, the correct application of these techniques and a continuous training of these therapists must be essential.

Keywords: dry needling, acupuncture, injection, adverse effect, safety

1. Introduction

Muscular pain is a very common pathology in the physiotherapy treatment of outpatient care. The invasive techniques for treating these patients have aroused great interest, there are many reviews made in recent years about its effectiveness but none with conclusive results [1–6]. Articles about post-needling pain [7, 8] and adverse side effects that may occur due to dry needling are being published until this day.

Dry needling is a minimally invasive technique into the most hypersensitive area/point of a tense band in a skeletal muscle (called myofascial trigger point), without the addition of any drug (**Figure 1**). It can be classified as deep or superficial [9]. There is not much evidence about which of the two options is better, it seems that deep dry needling has shown greater effectiveness due to penetrating the myofascial trigger point while the superficial dry needling penetrates the skin and the subcutaneous cellular tissue [10, 11]. In the same way, the appearance of local twitch response would guarantee its effectiveness [12, 13].

These myofascial trigger points present a high equivalence with the ashi points of acupuncture, corresponding to approximately 71% as Melzack introduced [14]. Acupuncture is based on a traditional and invasive Chinese technique of thousand years of age based on metaphysical concepts of "Ch'i" (Qi), the body energy flows through channels called "meridians" that has hypersensitive areas called ashi points

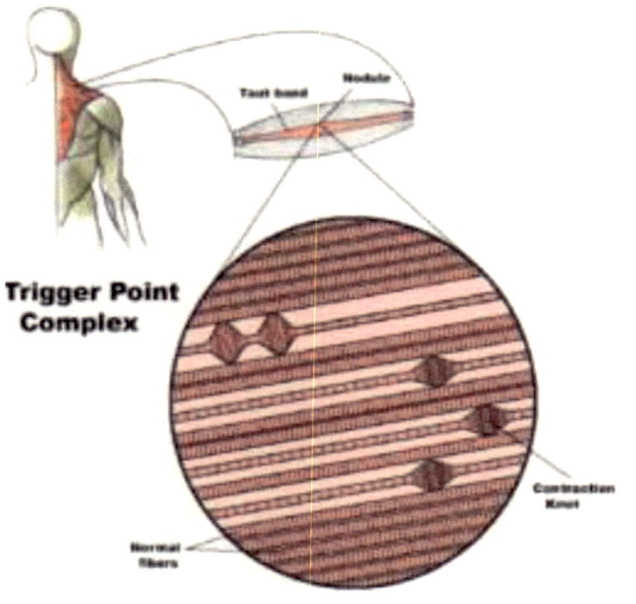

Figure 1.
Myofascial trigger point.

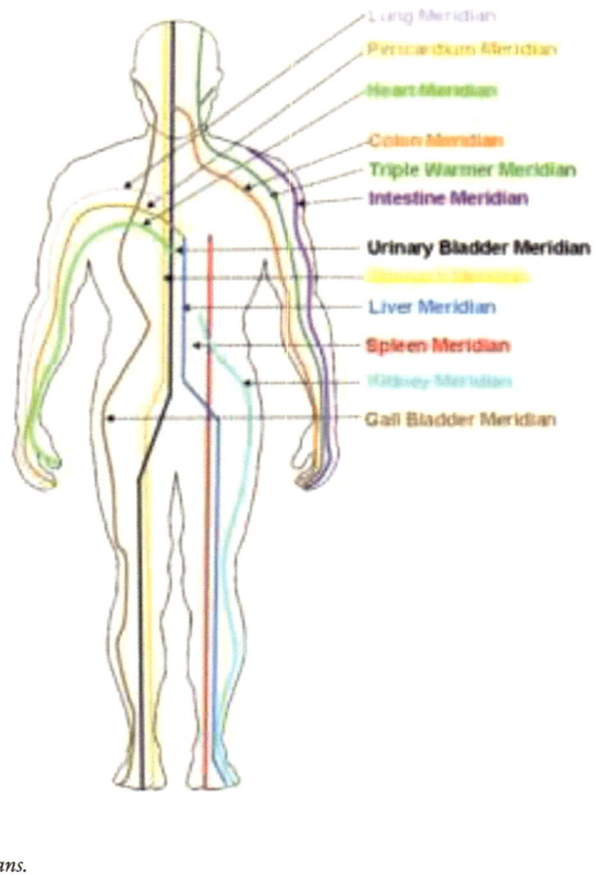

Figure 2.
Acupuncture Meridians.

(**Figure 2**). Its treatment also consists in the insertion of a needle in these points without any type of drugs [15].

On the other hand, injections have also been the subject of many reviews, [16, 17] they have combined the effects of needling with the effect of local anesthetics. However, in 1943 Lewit [18] demonstrated that the true effectiveness of the infiltrations was due to the mechanical effect generated by the insertion of the needle itself and not the anesthetic.

The objective of this study is to summarize the articles published in relation to adverse effects of needling therapies to promote a good practice and knowledge.

2. Method

2.1 Data sources and searches

A review of the literature was carried out in Pubmed, Web of Science, Medline and PEDro databases. The search was limited to studies on adverse effects and possible complications due to invasive/needling techniques: acupuncture, injections and dry needling in English and Spanish.

The keywords in English first introduced separately were: "acupuncture", "injection", "dry needling" and "adverse effect/event". In a second time, in order to limit the article sample, 12 searches were added: 1–3: "acupuncture/dry needling/injection" AND "complication"; 4–6: "acupuncture/dry needling/injection" AND "iatrogenic"; 7–9: "acupuncture/dry needling/injection" AND "safe practice" and 10–12: "acupuncture/dry needling/injection" AND "academic training". A manual search of the references of pre-selected articles was also carried out.

The search fields were title/abstract of the keywords of the studies publishes by the journals indexed in Pubmed during the period between 2000 (January) AND 2020 (January). In Web of Science the search fields were TS (theme)/TI (title). In Medline search field was TI (title) and in PEDro a simple search was done. The manuscripts selected for this systematic review met the following inclusion criteria: (i) articles that report the adverse effects and/or complications of invasive/needling techniques; (ii) reviews of such complications; (iii) articles in English and Spanish and (iv) articles with protocols or recommendations on the safe practice of these techniques. We excluded theoretical articles on the application of these techniques and articles that were not published in English or Spanish.

2.2 Study selection and data extraction

Type of articles: randomized clinical trials, case reports and reviews were included in this review. Letters to editor, commentaries to other articles and practical application of these techniques were excluded.

Type of participants: participants of all ages/nationalities/sex/gender/education level/socioeconomic status which has been treated with needling therapies.

Type of interventions and outcomes: articles which have reported adverse effects (mild-severe) due to acupuncture, dry needling and injection were selected.

Type of publications: full text articles published in English or Spanish. Once the articles were found, randomized clinical trials, case reports and reviews were selected. Once duplicates were removed, 2 reviewers analyzed the abstracts in a first screening and then carried out an exhaustive reading of the preselected ones until obtaining the final sample of articles reviewed and included in this study. If there was disagreement among the independent reviewers, a third reviewer decided. The data were extracted independently by the reviewers.

Data extraction: tables summarize the different adverse effects in chronological order classified in relation of the type of intervention.

Quality assessment: both authors selected, reviewed and assessed the quality of studies included in this review. Discrepancies were resolved by consensus.

2.3 Data synthesis and analysis

A summary of the findings of the included studies was performed, structured in the incidence/frequency of adverse effects, most prevalent adverse effects, type of intervention, type of population and other associated diseases which could influence the results (**Tables 1–3**). Each article was named by the author and date; they have a brief description of the intervention, the type of the adverse effect and the conclusion/resolution of the inconvenience.

3. Results

3.1 Selection of the studies

The initial search provided 4.034 potential reports, after applying the inclusion and exclusion criteria, the sample consisted of 2.169 articles from Pubmed, 814 articles from Web of Science, 781 articles from Medline, 270 from PEDro and 9

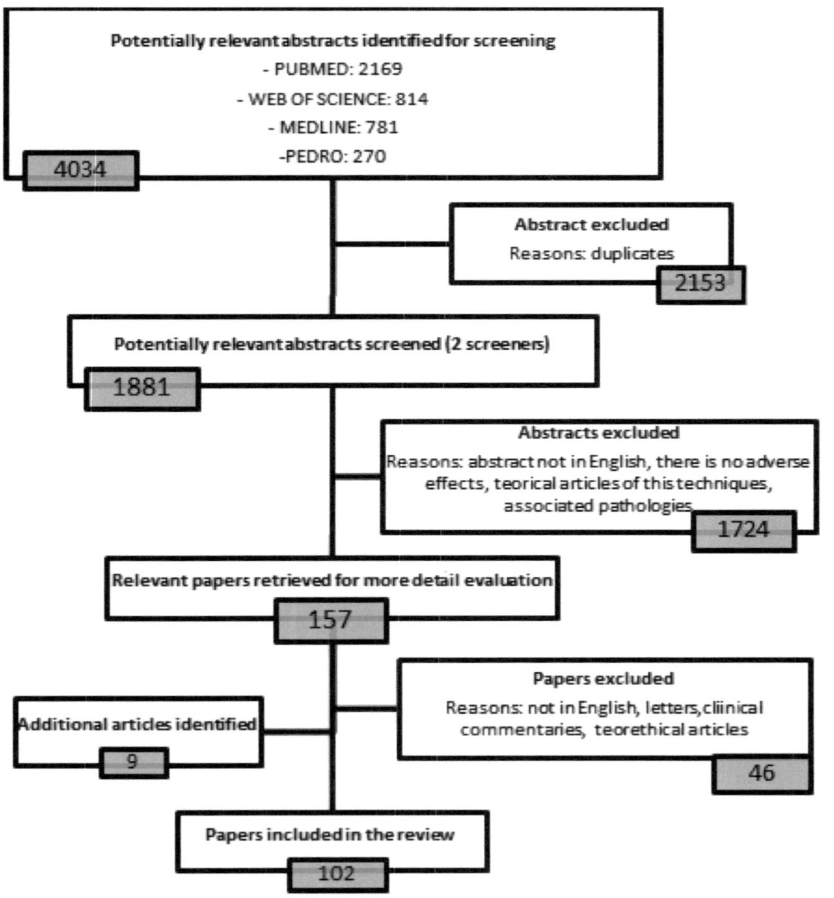

Figure 3.
Flow chart for different stages of the review.

found manually through preselected references from the Google Scholar database (**Figure 3**). After duplicated were excluded, 1.881 articles were selected. Both reviewers screened abstracts in a first time. In a second time, articles selected had a more detailed evaluation and 46 articles were excluded by the language, being letters to the editor or comments on other articles. Finally, 102 articles considered valid (93 from the initial search and 9 found manually). Detailed characteristics of the included studies are described in **Tables 1–3** in relation to acupuncture, injection or dry needling respectively.

Author/year	Description
Tandon, S. (1998) [19]	48-year-old male suffering from bronchial asthma. Pneumothorax following acupuncture with electrical stimulation in the third and fourth intercostal spaces.
Peuker, ET. (1999) [20]	To review the traumatic injuries after acupuncture and discuss how to avoid these adverse effects.
Kirchgatterer, A. (2000) [21]	83-year-old female. Syncope and cardiogenic shock after acupuncture into the sternum.
Lao, L. (2003) [22]	1965-1999 review: 202 incidents in 98 papers from 22 countries.
Ha, KY. (2003) [23]	68-year-old female. Low back pain and sciatica aggravated by acupuncture. Chronic inflammatory granuloma with compression of the lumbar fourth nerve and dural sac.
Chang, SA. (2004) [24]	68-year-old male. Death for massive hematemesis resulting from aortoduodenal fistula caused by acupuncture.
Saw, A.(2004) [25]	55-year-old female, diabetic. Necrotising fasciitis due to acupuncture in a knee osteoarthritis.
Lee, WM. (2005) [26]	36-year-old female. Bilateral pneumothorax after acupuncture.
Ryu, HJ. (2005) [27]	Clinical manifestations and treatment for Mycobacterium abscessus due to acupuncture.
Kung, YY. (2005) [28]	2 elderly patients: 72-year-old male and 63-year-old female. Between 2000 and 2002: syncope after acupuncture.
Chauffe, RJ. (2006) [29]	Since 1985: 9 pneumothorax cases after acupuncture. 27-year-old student seeking acupuncture at levator scapular.
Su, J. (2007) [30]	52-year-old female with chronic coughing. Acupuncture at BL131: paravertebral point at the level of the spinous process of the third vertebra: bilateral pneumothorax.
Lee, S. (2008) [31]	79-year-old male (hypertension and diabetes). Bacterial aortitis with pseudoaneurysm formation after acupuncture.
Hwang, JK. (2008) [32]	25-year-old female: Pneumoretroperitoneumen after acupuncture in right psoas muscle.
Juss, JK. (2008) [33]	50-year-old female. Pneumothorax by acupuncture at scapulothoracic region.
Jindal, V. (2008) [34]	Acupuncture to prevent postoperative nausea in children and to inhibit chemotherapy vomiting in adults.
Tsukazaki, Y. (2008) [35]	32-year-old female (recurrent headache). Subarachnoid hemorrhage following acupuncture.
Witt, CM. (2009) [36]	Review of acupuncture for osteoarthritis knee or hip, low back pain, neck pain or headache, asthma, rinitis or dysmenorrhoea. 229.230 patients: 19.726 suffered at least one adverse effect.
Kim, JH. (2009) [37]	55-year-old female. Hemopericardium after acupuncture.
Kuo, HF. (2010) [38]	39-year-old female with paresthesia and soreness at popliteal fossa. Fistula arteriovenous: vascular complication after acupuncture.

Author/year	Description
Ernst, E. (2010) [39]	Systematic review of cardiac tamponade due to acupuncture. 5 Databases, no restrictions in time or language. 26 cases (14 fatal consequences).
Nam, KH. (2010) [40]	4 cases of epidural hematomas after facet block, acupuncture and epidural injections.
Inayama, M. (2011) [41]	37-year-old female. Pneumothorax and pleural fluid collection after acupuncture on neck and upper back.
Hsieh, RL. (2011) [42]	44-year-old female (aplastic anemia). Staphylococcus infection after acupuncture at right calf.
He, W. (2012) [43]	Chinese review of 167 papers: 1.038 cases (35 deaths).
Xu, S. (2012) [44]	Frequency and severity of adverse events of acupuncture, moxibustion and cupping between 2000-11: 117 reports with 308 adverse effects from 25 countries.
Lee, JH. (2012) [45]	47-year-old female: epidural abscess at C1-C3 after acupuncture and cupping.
Tagami, R. (2013) [46]	69-year-old male: bilateral pneumothorax after acupuncture at upper back.
Stenger, M. (2013) [47]	64-year-old male: pneumothorax after acupuncture for lumbar pain and sciatica.
	82-year-old female: pneumothorax after acupuncture for herpes zoster.
Lee, SW. (2014) [48]	47-year-old female with abdominal pain after acupuncture. Endoscopy: needle in the posterior wall of the antrum.
Hamptom, DA. (2014) [49]	43-year-old female with chronic neck pain. Pneumothorax after acupuncture.
Peuker, E. (2014) [50]	38-year-old female. Pneumothorax after acupuncture at subacromial region (BL13), paravertebral point at the spinous process of the third thoracic vertebrae.
Chun, KJ. (2014) [51]	48-year-old female, (breast cancer 7 years before). Cardiac tamponade after acupuncture at fourth intercostal space.
Peuker, E. (2014) [52]	Review of traumatic lesions after acupuncture.
Wu, J. (2014) [53]	Chinese review of adverse effects between 1980 and 2013. 3 databases: 182 incidents in 133 relevant papers.
Ji, GY. (2014) [54]	54-year-old female; 38-year-old female and 60-year-old male: 3 cases of hemiplegia after cervical paraespinal needling (intramuscular stimulation, acupuncture or lidocaine) in 2002-2013 in Korea.
Schar, ML. (2015) [55]	39-year-old female with peripheral neuropathy history. Pneumothorax and broken needle in her chest.
Karavis, MY. (2015) [56]	37-year-old female. Haemothorax after acupuncture for neck and right upper back pain.
Callan, AK. (2015) [57]	15-year-old female with scoliosis. Periscapular abscess after acupuncture due to instrumentation.
White, A (2015) [58]	715 adverse effects: 90 trauma (186 secondary reports); 204 infections (91 reports); 144 miscellaneous (12 deaths).
Brogan, RJ. (2015) [59]	66-year-old male. Left pneumothorax after acupuncture (paraespinal, infrascapular and axillary regions bilaterally) for low back pain secondary to arthritis.
Wigger, O. (2015) [60]	51-year-old female with breast pain and dyspnea. Cardiac perforation due to acupuncture.

Author/year	Description
Yao, Y. (2015) [61]	54-year-old male. Epidural abscess at C4-T2 due to acupuncture.
Huisma, F. (2015) [62]	53-year-old female. Pneumothorax after acupuncture at posterior left hemithorax medial to the scapula.
Kim, JS. (2016) [63]	Review between 2011 and 2015: 17 pneumothoraxes (1 bilateral and 16 unilateral).
Ehgbal, K. (2016) [64]	74-year-old female. Quadriparesis and sensory deficit due to cervical subdural hematoma at C4-C6 after acupuncture at neck and shoulder.
Li, X. (2017) [65]	Meta-analysis of 33 randomized controlled trials about dry needling and manual acupuncture until February 2016. 33 trials with 1.692 patients.
Kim, D. (2017) [66]	55-year-old female. She died by acute peritonitis three days after acupuncture.
Domenicucci, M. (2017) [67]	64-year-old male. Hematoma epidural spinal C2-T12 (hemiparesis and paresthesias) after acupuncture for lumbosciatic pain.
Lee, HJ. (2017) [68]	Retrospective observational study (2010-2014): 10 pneumothorax and 2 pneumoperitoneum.
Sia, CH. (2018) [69]	50-year-old women. Pneumothorax after acupuncture for neck pain.
Lin, SK. (2019) [70]	Pneumothorax incidence after acupuncture in Taiwan (1997-2012) 411.734 patients, 5.407.378 treatments.
Lee, H. (2019) [71]	80-year-old male. Retroperitoneal abscess after lumbar acupuncture.
Lin, SK. (2019) [72]	Cellulitis after acupuncture incidence in Taiwan (1997-2012). 407.80 patients, 6.207.378 treatments.
Liu, ZH. (2019) [73]	42-year-old male. Broken needle in retroperitoneum after acupuncture treatments 2 years ago.
Tucciarone, M. (2019) [74]	36-year-old male. Abscess in prevertebral muscles after acupuncture.
Ullah, W. (2019) [75]	Old man. Pericarditis secondary to acupuncture after Staphilococus aureus infection.
Priola, SM. (2019) [76]	47-year-old female. Epidural intracraneal abscess after acupuncture.
Ullah, W. (2019) [77]	Systematic review about cardiac complications after acupuncture. 30 articles: 8 infections, 22 cardiac tamponades.
Corado, SC. (2019) [78]	79-year-old female. Pneumothorax 2 days after interscapular acupuncture.

Table 1.
Detail of articles included about acupuncture.

Author/year	Description
Antoni, RO. (1961) [79]	Review of 226 cases between 1955 and 1959: 71 iatrogenic pneumothoraxes.
Shafer, N. (1970) [80]	29-year-old female with severe neck pain with radiation into her right arm and limitation of motion. Pneumothorax after injection.
Cheng, J. (2007) [81]	Review from 1966 to November 2006: 35 papers. Infections, nerve injury, pneumothorax, embolism.
Usman, F. (2011) [82]	37-year-old female, 20 weeks pregnant. Retrosternal abscess after injection at sternoclavicular joint.
Ahiskalioglu, EO. (2016) [83]	25-year-old female. Pneumothorax after 4ml injection of lidocaine at thoracic region for neck and low back pain.

Author/year	Description
Soriano, PK. (2017) [84]	39-year-old male. Hipokalemic paralisis after injection guided by ultrasound in iliopsoas.
Choe, JY. (2017) [85]	70-year-old male (diabetic and cardiac history). Descending necrotizing mediastinitis after lidocaine injection at upper trapezius. Death by septic shock.
Lee, DG. (2018) [86]	38-year-old male. Scapular neuropathy after 1% lidocaine injection and 6ml of saline.
De la Torre-Canales, G. (2019) [87]	Systematic review about adverse effects of botulinum toxin A for masticatory muscles. 16 articles.
Camões-Barbosa, A. (2019) [88]	33-year-old female. Weakness after botulinum toxin A injection for spasticity.
Mozafari, N. (2019) [89]	55-year-old male. Cutaneous necrotic lesion after interferon beta 1-b injection.
Yurük, D. (2019) [90]	Rhabdomyolysis after epidural steroid injection.
Marcus, F. (2019) [91]	4 cases of Nicolau Syndrome: rare complication after intramuscular injections.
Kang, HY. (2019) [92]	Systemic toxicity after cervical epidural steroid injection guided (February 2016-October 2017) 11 patients.
Park, HB. (2019) [93]	Possible association between injections and calcification in lateral epicondylitis.
Al-Omari, AA. (2019) [94]	78-year-old male. Avascular necrosis after one intra-articular injection.
Lobaton, GO. (2019) [95]	62-year-old male. Vertebral osteomyelitis after epidural steroid injection. Permanent neurological injury.
Quincer, E. (2019) [96]	5-year-old male. Nicolau Syndrome after intramuscular injection in deltoid muscle.
Anderson, SE. (2019) [97]	Adverse effects after intra-articular corticosteroid injections (2000-2016), 1.708 patients, 104 adverse effects.
Kim, BR. (2019) [98]	Review of adverse events of intra-articular facet joint injections. (2007-2017). 11.980 procedures, 101 adverse events in 99 patients.
Wang, RN. (2019) [99]	61-year-old female. Oculo-motor nerve palsy after epidural lumbar injection.
Petrin, Z. (2019) [100]	87-year-old female. Paralysis without hematoma after lumbar epidural steroid injection.
Rensma, HG. (2019) [101]	33-year-old male. Nicolau syndrome after elbow injection.
Hu, Y. (2019) [102]	Optic perineuritis after hyaluronic acid injections.
Lee, JH. (2019) [103]	81-year-old female. Osteonecrosis after intra-articular corticosteroid injection.
Ali, D. (2019) [104]	72-year-old female. Ischaemic stroke after cervical transforaminal injection.
Rouientan, A. (2019) [105]	22-year-old male. Complication after botulinum toxin A.
Jani, P. (2019) [106]	Iatrogenic adrenal suppression after facet joint injection.
Desai, K. (2019) [107]	Review of 354 cases about iatrogenic peripheral nerve injuries.
Park, CW. (2019) [108]	68-year-old male. Iatrogenic injury of sciatic nerve after intramuscular injections.

Author/year	Description
Ali, SS. (2019) [109]	Iatrogenic spinal epidural hematoma and intracranial hypotension after thoracic epidural injection.
Sencan, S. (2019) [110]	3 males treated with transsacral blocks. Neuropatic sciatic after gluteal injection.

Table 2.
Detail of articles included about injections.

Author/year	Description
Lee, JH. (2011) [111]	58-year-old female with neck and upper extremity pain. Acute cervical epidural hematoma (C3-T1) after dry needling.
McCutcheon, L. (2011) [112]	Techniques modifications to avoid pleura and lung. Understanding anatomy and its variants. Safe technique for training physiotherapists.
Brady, S. (2014) [113]	2 questionnaires for 10 months. 39 physiotherapists and 1463 adverse effects. Safe technique.
Halle, JS. (2016) [114]	To evaluate benefits/risks of these techniques to minimize them.
Halle, JS. (2016) [115]	Adequate training and education: safe and effective technique. To inform patients via informed consent.
McManus, R. (2018) [116]	27-year-old female, secretary. Neurapraxia of radial nerve after dry needling.
Berrigan, WA. (2018) [117]	62-year-old female. Epidural hematoma and broken needle after dry needling.
Uzar, T. (2018) [118]	36-year-old male. Pneumothorax after dry needling for pain in back muscles.
Kim, DC. (2018) [119]	16-year-old male. Local abscess after dry needling at the thigh for pain after a knee injury.
McDowell, JM. (2018) [120]	Safety of acupuncture and dry needling in pregnant women. 124 responses: only 60 needle pregnant women and a 60% of them feel safety.

Table 3.
Detail of articles included about dry needling.

3.2 Characteristics of the reviewed articles

102 articles met the inclusion criteria of the research in the period between 2000 (January) and 2020 (January) in form of original articles, case reports and reviews.

From these 102 articles selected, 23 refer to pneumothorax including more than 120 cases (19 of acupuncture, 3 of injection and 2 of dry needling); 4 articles refer to cardiac tamponade with more than 25 cases (both of acupuncture), 21 in relation to infections, abscesses or hemorrhages (14 of acupuncture, 6 of injection and 1 of dry needling) and other 7 articles refer to adverse effects such as syncope and cardiogenic shock (acupuncture), 3 pneumoperitoneo (acupuncture), 9 hematoma (6 of acupuncture, 1 of injection, 2 of dry needling), hemiplegia (acupuncture), cardiac perforation (acupuncture), hypokalemic paralysis (injection), 6 neuropathies (injection), 1 neuroapraxia (dry needling) and 12 cutaneous lesions/Nicolau syndrome/necrosis (3 of acupuncture, 9 of injection). In 11 articles there already was an existing disease, in other 4 the needle was broken and unfortunately in 4 articles the consequences were fatal. It has also collected 21 review articles of these needling therapies (more than 21.000 adverse effects described). Finally, 6 articles have synthetized information about benefits, risks, perception of security and even modifications of the application of these techniques (**Figure 4**).

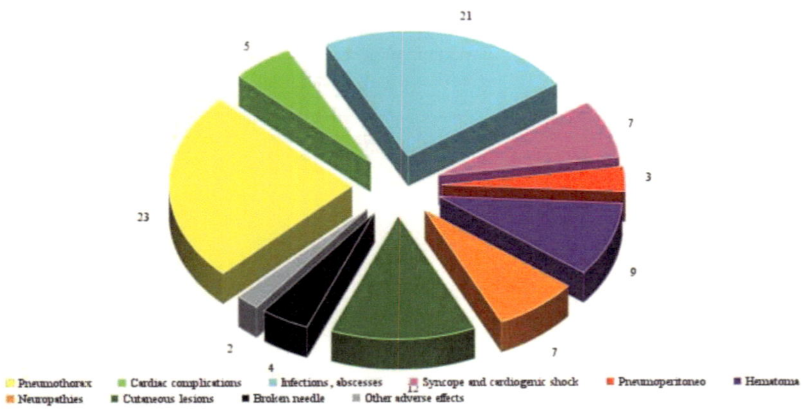

Figure 4.
Prevalence of most common adverse events.

4. Discussion

Considering the outpatient care treatment, adverse effects are possible complications that can occur during or even after the application of these techniques. In more cases there has little importance such as pain, a slight bleeding or a small bruise that disappears quickly. However, other adverse effects without a clear cause can suppose a serious risk for the patient.

These risks have always been present, but in recent years publications have increased considerably. There is no consensus about the classification of these adverse effects. Some authors [111] categorized them into four groups: delayed or missed diagnosis, adverse effects during treatment, bacterial or viral infections, or tissue or organ trauma.

4.1 Incidence/frequency of adverse effects

The incidence/frequency of these adverse effects is not clear. Acupuncture seems to have an incidence of 2/125.000 cases [30]; White et al. [58] estimated the risk of a serious adverse event with acupuncture at 0.05 per 10.000 treatments, and 0.55 per 10.000 individual patients, Lin et al. [70] reported a pneumothorax incidence of 0.87 per 1.000.000 acupuncture treatments and 1.75 per 1.000.000 in anatomical risk areas; these authors also showed a cellulitis incidence [72] about 64.4 per 100.000 treatments.

In relation to injections, Anderson et al. [97] explained an incidence of 5.8% of adverse effects. Kim et al. [93] introduced the incidence separately in relation with the case: 0.84% and 1.63% in relation to the patient; on the other hand, the procedure had an incidence of 0.07% and the administrated drug 0.15%. Finally, the unknown etiology had a 0.63% for this author [93] and for other authors it is unknown [121].

Data about incidence of dry needling procedures has not been found.

The most reviewed articles refer isolated cases and not a periodicity, but other authors have published several reviews that try to synthesize this information. Considering these 3 needling techniques, acupuncture leaves a clear superiority in relation to the number of publications with adverse effects.

Peuker et al. [20] investigated the traumatic wounds caused by acupuncture and discuss how these complications could be avoided. Lao et al. [22] reviewed 98 publications (1965–1999) and they found 202 complications (infections, tissue/organ damage and nerve injury). Cutaneous disorders, hypotension, fainting and vomiting were some adverse effects described. Chauffe et al. [29] found 9 cases of pneumothorax since 1985. Witt et al. [36] reviewed acupuncture studies in chronic osteoarthritis pain of the knee or hip, lumbar, cervical, head, allergic rhinitis, dysmenorrhea and asthma. Out of 229.230, 19.726 reported at least 1 adverse effect (bleeding, pain, vegetative symptoms). The longest duration of these adverse effects was 180 days (nerve injury). Ernst et al. [39] conducted a review of cardiac tamponade after acupuncture: 26 cases were found and 14 with fatal complications. He et al. [43] reviewed 167 articles with 1.038 cases (35 deaths) from Chinese literature. 468 cases were syncope, 307 pneumothorax, and 64 subarachnoid hemorrhage. Xu et al. [44] checked the frequency and severity of these effects (2000–2011): 117 articles with 308 adverse effects in 25 countries (294 for acupuncture, 4 moxibustion and 10 cupping). Peuker et al. [52] reviewed the traumatic lesions after acupuncture. Wu et al. [53] performed a review in China (1980–2013), finding 182 incidents in 133 papers (internal organ, tissue and nerve injury are the major complications). The adverse effects included were syncope, infection, hemorrhage, allergy, burn, aphonia, hysteria, cough, thirst, fever, somnolence and broken needles. White et al. [58] found 715 incidents in their review: 90 reports of trauma and 12 reports of death. In Taiwan, Lin et al. [70, 72] published 2 reviews (1997–2012) about pneumothorax and cellulitis incidence respectively. They evaluated 411.734 patients with 5.407.378 treatments of acupuncture [70] and 407.802 patients with 6.207.378 acupuncture treatments [72]. In both articles the authors emphasized the importance of the previous medical history. Ullah et al. [77] reviewed 133 articles and selected 30 cases with relevant cardiac complications: 8 were infective complications and 22 cardiac tamponades.

Regarding injections, 8 articles have been found. Antoni Ro et al. [79] reviewed 226 cases (1955–1959), finding 71 cases of pneumothorax and Cheng et al. [81] performed a review (1966–2006) explaining the complications of this technique: "infections, spinal cord injury and peripheral nerve injuries, pneumothorax, air embolism, pain or swelling at the site of injection, chemical meningism, granulomatous inflammation of the synovium, aseptic acute arthritis, embolia cutis medicamentosa, skeletal muscle toxicity, and tendon and fascial ruptures". De la Torre et al. [87] introduced a review about the adverse effects caused by botulinum toxin A in masticatory muscles. They used 436 citations and concluded with 16:7 were myofascial pain and 9 were trigeminal neuralgia. The most frequent adverse effects were "temporary regional weakness, tenderness over the injection sites and minor discomfort during chewing". Most of them had a spontaneous resolution. Marcus et al. [91] found a very rare complication due to injections (diclofenac, dexamethasone and benzathine penicilin): Nicolau Syndrome. They found 4 cases (2016–2018). Park et al. [93] investigates an association between steroid injection and calcification in lateral epicondylitis. They evaluated 110 patients (February 2016-October 2018) and concluded that the injections history and the number of them has a significative association with soft tissue calcifications. A review (January 2000-April 2016) about adverse events due to intra-articular corticosteroid injections was made by Anderson et al. [97] 1.708 patients from 3 regional hospital participated: 99 patients had 104 adverse effects within 90 days post-injection. The most prevalent symptom was flare (78 patients) and 10 patients had skin reactions. There were no infections. Years before, Kim et al. [98] had reviewed 11.980 injections in 6.066 patients (January 2007-December 2017). There were 101 facet-joint injections and 99 patients developed adverse effects. 7 patients had an infectious spondylitis, 1 patient died of an uncontrolled infection and 2 patients had partial recovery of their neurological condition. Finally, Desai et al. [107] published a review of 17 years where reflected the iatrogenic peripheral nerve injuries due to injections. They included "intramuscular injections, brachial nerves procedures, subclavian and jugular venous cannulation and routine intravenous injections". The most frequents symptoms were pain, paresthesia and sensory-motor deficits. 190 patients needed surgical intervention, 164 had any sequel or no recovery and 9 had neurological deterioration with weakness.

There is not standard data on the incidence of these events. Unfortunately, the huge diversity of pathologies, interventions, therapists... makes difficult a generalization.

4.2 Most prevalent adverse effects

There is no consensus about the most frequent adverse effect in the literature. Some of them are pneumothorax, cardiac tamponade, air embolism, spinal epidural haematoma/abscess, abdominal visceral injury, median and fibular nerve injury and infection [20, 36, 75, 77, 81, 87, 111].

Some authors reflected that pneumothorax is the most cited adverse effect, [50, 63] while for others is infection [44]. White et al. [58] agree with both theories being the most common complication pneumothorax and injury to the central nervous system and infection will be in second place. Ullah et al. [77] concluded that cardiac tamponade is the most frequent complication.

It seems that invasive techniques on the thorax are related to a high incidence of pneumothorax [118]. There are some investigations in different countries (United Kingdom, Japan, Czechoslovakia, Switzerland, Germany, Japan and Taiwan) about it. The incidence of these cases is low, less than 1/10.000. However, there have been more than 100 cases reporting iatrogenic pneumothorax due to acupuncture and dry needling, including cases of death [112]. Lin et al. [70] showed an incidence of 0.84/1.000.000 and 1,75/1.000.000 at risk anatomical areas. Most iatrogenic pneumothorax used to be unilateral, but there are bilateral cases too [26, 30]. In this article there are 23 articles related to pneumothorax [19, 26, 29, 30, 33, 46, 47, 49, 50, 55, 56, 59, 62, 63, 68–70, 78–80, 83, 112, 118].

Other incidents (less frequent) reported in the literature but not less important are cardiac tamponade [21, 39, 51, 75, 77], granulomas [23], fistulas [24, 38], necrosis [25, 42, 85], infections [27, 57, 119], abscesses [27, 45, 61, 71, 74, 76], pneumoretroperitoneum [32], hemorrhages [35], hemopericardium [37], haematomas [40, 64, 67, 109, 111, 117], chilotorax [41], organ perforation [48, 60], needle rupture [53, 55, 117], hemiplegia [54], hemothorax [56], peritonitis [66], cellulitis [72], hypokalemic paralysis [84], nerve injury [86, 99, 102, 107, 108, 110, 116], weakness [88], necrosis [89, 90, 94, 103], Nicolau Sydrome [91, 96, 101], toxicity...[92] Almost all had a complete resolution of the symptoms. However, publications with fatal and irreversible consequences have also been found [24, 37, 98].

4.3 Special considerations

There are several aspects must be considered when carrying out these techniques in the treatment of muscular pain in outpatients. These incidents, even taking caution may occur; therefore, it is important to obtain a complete clinical history highlighting possible underlying pathologies [70–72]. Several articles have found patients with asthma [19], diabetes [25, 85], anemia [42], herpes zoster [47], cancer [51], miastenia gravis [55] and scoliosis [57] and sclerosis [89]. These pathologies could influence the appearance or greater probability of developing a complication.

4.4 Type of population

The age of the patients is other aspect to discuss. A review performed in children (acupuncture to prevent postoperative nausea) has been published without conclusion about its effectiveness [34]. Quincer et al. [96] showed the case of a 5-year-old boy who developed a Nicolau Syndrome after an intramuscular injection in deltoid. Besides, cases of elderly people who have suffered syncope's due to acupuncture have also been described [28]. These patients (the most prevalent population in the outpatient) may be more debilitated and suffer more adverse effects even taking precautions.

There are some types of population could be considered "at risk" when using these needling techniques, like pregnant women. We have found an article that exposes a retrosternal abscess due to sternoclavicular joint injection with resolution [82]. McDowell et al. have developed a review on the safety of acupuncture and dry needling in pregnant women in New Zealand. They conclude that of 124 responses obtained, only 60 therapists needle pregnant women and only 66% of them express safety. More training is needed in this field, particularly on dry needling [120].

In relation to sex, only one article showed major incidence in men than in woman [70].

4.5 Other applications of needling therapies

It seems that the most frequent application of these techniques is analgesia, including analgesic blocks [40], but there are other applications such hyaluronic acid in eyebrow [102], botulinum toxin A for axilar hiperhidrosis [105] and aesthetics for rejuvenation have also presented adverse effects [122, 123].

4.6 Reviews about safety

Among all reviews a meta-analysis of 33 randomized controlled trials was found. The authors conclude that acupuncture and dry needling are effective techniques, but more research on the safety of them is needed [65]. McCutcheon et al. [112] also reviewed the safety of acupuncture and dry needling, suggesting modifications of these techniques to avoid pleura and the lung. However, there are no conclusive results.

Considering the severity of these techniques, Brady et al. [113] conducted a study to check the adverse effects of dry needling. They filled in 2 questionnaires for 10 months to 39 physiotherapists and regrouped 1.463 adverse effects (common/less common/rare). They showed that it was a safe technique. Similarly, Halle et al. have published 2 articles [114, 115]. They assessed the risk/benefit of these techniques to minimize them, proposed an adequate education, knowledge of anatomy, training and to inform the patient via informed consent.

Guided techniques should be an interesting option to reduce these complications, but several articles do not support this affirmation [92, 110]. More investigation in this line is needed. On the other side, if dry needling seems to be safe, maybe it would be chosen instead injections to avoid the possible events effects derivate to the administered drugs like Kim et al. [93] exposed.

4.7 Limitations

Language was the first limitation, several articles have been found in France [124, 125], Portugal [126], Russia [127], Germany [128], Italy [129], Denmark [130], and Iceland [131] that have not been included in the revision due to its original language. 3 reviews in Chinese [132], German [128] and Danish [133] respectively were excluded for the same reason. The first two expose a synthesis or classification of adverse effects and the third, is a review on acupuncture in children in Denmark. Letters and comments were also excluded; however, we highlight the case of acupuncture in the disease of behgets [134]; a letter to editor where they expose a case of pneumothorax during a demonstration of dry needling in the thoracic iliocostal [135] and a needle broken as a complication of acupuncture [136]. Neither has been taken into account articles on practical applications, effectiveness of such techniques or superiority of some over others.

4.8 Future investigations

Acupuncture seems to have the most adverse effects reported throughout the literature, while injections and dry needling are increasing their publications, probably due to the increase in popularity especially of the second [114, 115]. Nowadays adverse effects seem to be common, but complications are rare. All authors of these articles agree in some tips to take in consideration:

- The anatomy of the area to treat should be familiar to the healthcare professionals before undertaking the procedure.
- Communication with the patient via informed consent is needed.
- Aseptic conditions during the procedure are necessary.
- The appropriate time to apply the treatments correctly becomes essential for a good practice and an adequate achievement of the results.
- A correct training and continuous formation of healthcare practitioners are necessary.

5. Conclusion

This is a brief summary of the adverse effects found in the literature. There is no clear consensus about incidence, the most prevalent adverse effect, the intervention protocols, or experience of the therapist... As a conclusion, needling therapies are usual techniques in the outpatient care and complications are possible even considering all the precautions. Therapists have to know how to react, recognize the adverse effects and correct them as far as possible or refer the patient to the corresponding service, being always updated to new advances and familiar to the normal and variants of anatomy of the patients to avoid complications as much as possible. Caring the aseptic conditions and the communication with the patient to inform them about all the parts of the treatment with needling therapies are essential.

Conflict of interest

None declared.

Author details

Inés Llamas-Ramos[1†] and Rocío Llamas-Ramos[1,2*†]

1 University of Salamanca, C/ Donantes de Sangre s/n, 37007, Salamanca, Spain

2 FREMAP, C/ Las Eras, esquina Pollo Martín, nº 11, 37005, Salamanca, Spain

*Address all correspondence to: rociollamas@usal.es

† Both authors equally contributed as first authors in the manuscript.

References

[1] Dunning J, Butts R, Mourad F, Young I, Flannagan S, Perreault T. Dry needling a literature review with implications for clinical practice guidelines. Phys Ther Rev. 2014 Aug;**19**(4):252-265

[2] Boyles R, Fowler R, Ramsey D, Burrows E. Effectiveness of trigger point dry needling for multiple body regions a systematic review. J Man Manip Ther. 2015 Dec;**23**(5):276-293

[3] Fogelman Y, Kent J. Efficacy of dry needling for treatment of myofascial pain syndrome. J Back Musculoskelet Rehabil. 2015;**28**(1):173-179

[4] Rodríguez-Mansilla J, González-Sánchez B, De Toro GÁ, Valera-Donoso E, Garrido-Ardila EM, Jiménez-Palomares M, et al. Effectiveness of dry needling on reducing pain intensity in patients with myofascial pain syndrome a Meta-analysis. J Tradit Chin Med. 2016 Feb;**36**(1):1-13

[5] Espejo-Antúnez L, Tejeda JF, Albornoz-Cabello M, Rodríguez-Mansilla J, de la Cruz-Torres B, Ribeiro F, et al. Dry needling in the management of myofascial trigger points. A systematic review of randomized controlled trials. Complement Ther Med. 2017 Aug;**33**:46-57

[6] Gattie E, Cleland JA, Snodgrass S. The effectiveness of trigger point dry needling for musculoskeletal conditions by physical therapists a systematic review and meta-analysis. J Orthop Sports Phys Ther. 2017 Mar;**47**(3):133-149

[7] Martín-Pintado-Zugasti A, Mayoral Del Moral O, Gerwin RD, Fernández-Carnero J. Post-needling soreness after myofascial trigger point dry needling. Current status and future research. J Bodyw Mov Ther. 2018 Oct;**22**(4):941-946

[8] Martín-Pintado-Zugasti A, Fernández-Carnero J, León-Hernández JV, Calvo-Lobo C, Beltran-Alacreu H, Alguacil-Diego I, Gallego-Izquierdo T, Pecos-Martin D. Postneedling soreness and tenderness after different dosages of dry needling of an active myofascial trigger point in patients with neck pain. A randomized controlled trial. PM R. 2018 May 29. pii: S1934-1482(18)30287-9.

[9] Travell JG, Simons DG. Myofascial pain and dysfunction: the trigger point manual. Vol. 1. Baltmore, MD: Williams & Wilkins; 1983

[10] Baldry P. Superficial versus deep dry needling. Acupunct Med. 2002 Aug;**20**(2-3):78-81

[11] Sedighi A, Nakhostin Ansari N, Naghdi S. Comparison of acute effects of superficial and deep dry needling into trigger points of suboccipital and upper trapezius muscles in patients with cervicogenic headache. J Bodyw Mov Ther. 2017 Oct;**21**(4):810-814

[12] Perreault T, Dunning J, Butts R. The local twitch response during trigger point dry needling Is it necessary for successful outcomes? J Bodyw Mov Ther. 2017 Oct;**21**(4):940-947

[13] Fernández-Carnero J, Gilarranz-de-Frutos L, León-Hernández JV, Pecos-Martin D, Alguacil-Diego I, Gallego-Izquierdo T, et al. Effectiveness of different deep dry needling dosages in the treatment of patients with cervical myofascial pain. A pilot RCT. Am J Phys Med Rehabil. 2017 Oct;**96**(10):726-733

[14] Melzack R, Stillwell DM, Fox EJ. Trigger points and acupuncture points

for pain: correlations and implications. Pain. 1977;**3**(1):3-23

[15] Ulett GA, Han S, Han JS. Electroacupuncture: mechanism and clinical application. Biological psychiatry. 1998;**44**(2):129-138

[16] Cox J, Varatharajan S, Côté P. Optima Collaboration. Effectiveness of Acupuncture Therapies to Manage Musculoskeletal Disorders of the Extremities A Systematic Review. J Orthop Sports Phys Ther. 2016 Jun;**46**(6):409-429

[17] Li X, Wang R, Xing X, Shi X, Tian J, Zhang J, et al. Acupuncture for Myofascial Pain Syndrome A Network Meta-Analysis of 33 Randomized Controlled Trials. Pain Physician. 2017 Sep;**20**(6):E883-E902

[18] Lewit K. The needle effect in the relief of myofascial pain. Pain. 1979;**6**(1):83-90

[19] Tandon S, Gupta KB. Acupuncture induced pneumothorax – a case report. Medical Journal of Indonesia. May 1998;**7**(2):111

[20] Peuker ET, White A, Ernst E, Pera F, Filler TJ. Traumatic complications of acupuncture. Therapists need to know human anatomy. Arch Fam Med. 1999 Nov-Dec;**8**(6):553-558

[21] Kirchgatterer A, Schwarz CD, Höller E, Punzengruber C, Hartl P, Eber B. Cardiac tamponade following acupuncture. Chest. 2000 May;**117**(5):1510-1511

[22] Lao L, Hamilton GR, Fu J, Berman BM. Is acupuncture safe? A systematic review of case reports. Altern Ther Health Med. 2003 Jan-Feb;**9**(1):72-83

[23] Ha KY, Kim YH. Chronic inflammatory granuloma mimics clinical manifestations of lumbar spinal stenosis after acupuncture: a case report. Spine (Phila Pa 1976). 2003 Jun 1;**28**(11):E217-E220

[24] Chang SA, Kim YJ, Sohn DW, Park YB, Choi YS. Aortoduodenal fistula complicated by acupuncture. Int J Cardiol. 2005 Sep 30;**104**(2):241-242

[25] Saw A, Kwan MK, Sengupta S. Necrotising fasciitis: a life-threatening complication of acupuncture in a patient with diabetes mellitus. Singapore Med J. 2004 Apr;**45**(4):180-182

[26] Lee WM, Leung HB, Wong WC. Iatrogenic bilateral pneumothorax arising from acupuncture: a case report. J Orthop Sur (Hong Kong). 2005 Dec;**13**(3):300-302

[27] Ryu HJ, Kim WJ, Oh CH, Song HJ. Iatrogenic Mycobacterium abscessus infection associated with acupuncture: clinical manifestations and its treatment. Int J Dermatol. 2005 Oct;**44**(10):846-850

[28] Kung YY, Chen FP, Hwang SJ, Hsieh JC, Lin YY. Convulsive syncope: an unusual complication of acupuncture treatment in older patients. J Altern Complement Med. 2005 Jun;**11**(3):535-537

[29] Chauffe RJ, Duskin AL. Pneumothorax secondary to acupuncture therapy. South Med J. 2006 Nov;**99**(11):1297-1299

[30] Su JW, Lim CH, Chua YL. Bilateral pneumothorax as a complication of acupuncture. Singapore Med J. 2007 Jan;**48**(1):e32-e33

[31] Lee S, Lim SH, Kim DK, Joo HC. Acupuncture induced necrotizing aortitis with infected pseudoaneurysm formation. Yonsei Med J. 2008 Apr 30;**49**(2):322-324

[32] Hwang JK, Kim J, Lee BJ, Park JJ, Kim JS, Bak YT.

Pneumoretroperitoneum following acupuncture. J Altern Complement Med. 2008 Dec;**14**(10):1299-1301

[33] Juss JK, Speed CA, Warrington J, Mahadeva R. Acupuncture induced pneumothorax – a case report. Acupunct Med. 2008 Sep;**26**(3):193-196

[34] Jindal V, Ge A, Mansky PJ. Safety and efficacy of acupuncture in children: a review of the evidence. J Pediatr Hematol Oncol. 2008 Jun;**30**(6):431-442

[35] Tsukazaki Y, Inagaki T, Yamanouchi Y, Kawamoto K, Oka N. Traumatic subarachnoid hemorrhage associated with acupuncture. Headache. 2008 Sep;**48**(8):1240-1241

[36] Witt CM, Pach D, Brinkhaus B, Wruck K, Tag B, Mank S, et al. Safety of acupuncture: results of a prospective observational study with 229.230 patients and introduction of a medical information and consent form. Forsch Komplementmed. 2009 Apr;**16**(2):91-97

[37] Kim JH, Kim S, Lee YJ, Ahn R, Hong ES. Hemopericardium following acupuncture. Yonsei Med J. 2011 Jan;**52**(1):207-209. DOI: 10.3349/ymj.2011.52.1.207

[38] Kuo HF, Shih MC, Kao WP, Su HM, Lin TH, Voon WC, et al. Acupuncture induced popliteal arteriovenous fistula successfully treated with percutaneous endovascular intervention. Kaohsiung J Med Sci. 2010 Mar;**26**(3):158-162

[39] Ernst E, Zhang J. Cardiac tamponade caused by acupuncture: a review of the literature. Int J Cardiol. 2011 Jun 16;**149**(3):287-289

[40] Nam KH, Choi CH, Yang MS, Kang DW. Spinal epidural hematoma after pain control procedure. J Korean Neurosurg Soc. 2010 Sep;**48**(3):281-284

[41] Inayama M, Shinohara T, Hino H, Yoshida M, Ogushi F. Chylothorax caused by acupuncture. Intern Med. 2011;**50**(20):2375-2377

[42] Hsieh RL, Huang CH, Uen WC. Necrotizing fasciitis after acupuncture in a patient with aplastic anemia. J Altern Complement Med. 2011 Sep;**17**(9):871-874

[43] He W, Zhao X, Li Y, Xi Q, Guo Y. Adverse events following acupuncture: a systematic review of the Chinese literature for the years 1956-2010. J Altern Complement Med. 2012 Oct;**18**(10):892-901

[44] Xu S, Wang L, Cooper E, Zhang M, Manheimer E, Berman B, et al. Adverse events of acupuncture: a systematic review of case reports. Evid Based Complement Alternat Med. 2013;**2013**:581203

[45] Lee JH, Cho JH, Jo DJ. Cervical epidural abscess after cupping and acupuncture. Complement Ther Med. 2012 Aug;**20**(4):228-231

[46] Tagami R, Moriya T, Kinoshita K, Tanjoh K. Bilateral tension pneumothorax related to acupuncture. Acupunct Med. 2013 Jun;**31**(2):242-244

[47] Stenger M, Bauer NE, Licht PB. Is pneumothorax after acupuncture so uncommon? J Thorac Dis. 2013 Aug;**5**(4):E144-E146

[48] Lee SW, Ahn JY, Choi WJ, Kim EJ, Bae SH, Choi YS, et al. A needle penetrating the stomach cavity after acupuncture. Clin Endosc. 2014 May;**47**(3):258-261

[49] Hampton DA, Kaneko RT, Simeon E, Moren A, Rowell S, Watters JM. Acupuncture-Related Pneumothorax. Med Acupunct. 2014 Aug 1;**26**(4):241-245

[50] Peuker E. Case report of tension pneumothorax related to acupuncture. Acupunct Me. 2004 Mar;**22**(1):40-43

[51] Chun KJ, Lee SG, Son BS, Kim DH. Life-threatening cardiac tamponade: a rare complication of acupuncture. J Cardiothorac Surg. 2014 Mar 31;**9**:61

[52] Peuker E, Grönemeyer D. Rare but serious complications of acupuncture: traumatic lesions. Acupunct med. 2001 Dec;**19**(2):103-108

[53] Wu J, Hu Y, Zhy Y, Yin P, Litscher G, Xu S. Systematic review of adverse effects: a further step towards modernization of acupuncture in China. Evid Based Complement Alternat Med. 2015;**2015**:432467

[54] Ji GY, Oh CH, Choi WS, Lee JB. Three cases of hemiplegia after cervical paraspinal muscle needling. Spine J. 2015 Mar 1;**15**(3):e9-e13

[55] Scharf ML, Kommuri A. delayed recognition of an uncommon cause of iatrogenic pneumothorax. J Bronchology Interv Pulmonol. 2015 Apr;**22**(2):162-164

[56] Karavis MY, Argyra E, Segredos V, Yiallouroy A, Giokas G, TheodosopoulosT. Acupuncture-induced haemothorax: a rare iatrogenic complication of acupuncture. Acupunct Med. 2015 Jun;**33**(3):237-241

[57] Callan AK, Bauer JM, Martus JE. Deep spine infection after acupuncture in the setting of spinal instrumentation. Spine Deform. 2016 Mar;**4**(2):156-161

[58] White A. A cumulative review of the range and incidence of significant adverse events associated with acupuncture. Acupunct Med. 2004 Sep;**22**(3):122-133

[59] Brogan RJ, Mushtaq F. Acupuncture-induced pneumothorax: the hidden complication. Scott Med J. 2015 May;**60**(2):e11-e13

[60] Wigger O, Stortecky S, Most H, Englberger L. Cardiac perforation as a rare complication of acupuncture. Eur Heart J. 2016 May 1;**37**(17):1383

[61] Yao Y, Hong W, Chen H, Guan Q, Yu H, Chang X, et al. Cervical spinal epidural abscess following acupuncture and wet cupping therapy: a case report. Complement Ther Med. 2016 Feb;**24**:108-110

[62] Huisma F, Konrad G, Thomas S. Pneumothorax after acupuncture. Can Fam Physician. 2015 Dec;**61**(12):1071-1073

[63] Kim JS, Kim KH, Kim WW. 17 cases of pneumothorax and factors influencing pneumothorax. Acupunct Electrother Res. 2016;**41**(2):95-105

[64] Eghbal K, Ghaffarpasand F. An acute cervical subdural hematoma as the complication of acupuncture: case report and literature review. World Neurosurg. 2016 Nov;95:616.e11-616.e13.

[65] Li X, Wang R, Xing X, Shi X, Tian J, Zhang J, et al. Acupuncture for myofascial pain syndrome: a network Meta-Analysis of 33 randomized controlled trials. Pain Physician. 2017 Sep;**20**(6):E883-E902

[66] Kim D, Lee S. An autopsy case of fatal acute peritonitis complicated by illegal acupuncture therapy. Forensic Sci Int. 2017 Jul;**276**:e13-e15

[67] Domenicucci M, Marruzzo D, Pesce A, Raco A, Missori P. Acute spinal epidural hematoma after acupuncture; personal case and literature review. World Neurosurg. 2017 Jun;102:695.e11-695.e14.

[68] Lee HJ, Kim YJ, Kim WY. Safety concerns with thoracoabdominal acupuncture: experience at a tertiary-care emergency department. Pain Med. 2017 Dec 1;**18**(12):2504-2508

[69] Sia CH, Leow AS, Leong BS. Traumatic pneumothorax secondary

to acupuncture needling. Cureus. 2018 Aug 23;**10**(8):e3194

[70] Lin SK, Liu JM, Hsu RJ, Chuang HC, Wang YX, Lin PH. Incidence of iatrogenic pneumothorax following acupuncture treatments in Taiwan. Acupunct Med. 2019 Dec;**37**(6):332-339

[71] Lee H, Sung K, Cho J. Retroperitoneal abscess with pylephlebitis caused by lumbar acupuncture: a case report. BMC Surg. 2019 Oct 16;**19**(1):145

[72] Lin SK, Liu JM, Wang PH, Hung SP, Hsu RJ, Chuang HC, Lin PH. Incidence of cellulitis following acupuncture treatments in Taiwan. Int J Environ Res Public Health. 2019 Oct 11;16(20). pii: E3831.

[73] Liu ZH, Wang HD, Xu X, Man LB. Removal of a broken acupuncture needle in retroperitoneum by laparoscopy: a case report. BMC Surg. 2019 Aug 6;**19**(1):102

[74] Tucciarone M, Taliente S, Gómez-Blasi Camacho R, Souviron Encabo R, González-Orús Á-MR. Extensive pyomyositis of prevertebral muscles after acupuncture: Case report. Turk J Emerg Med. 2019 Apr 4;**19**(3):113-114

[75] Ullah W, Roomi S, Sattar Z, Ahmad A, Ali Z, Sarwar U, et al. Acupuncture related acute purulent pericarditis masquerading uremic pericarditis. J Community Hosp Intern Med Perspect. 2019 Jun 19;**9**(3):230-234

[76] Priola SM, Moghaddamjou A, Ku JC, Taslimi S, Yang VXD. Acupuncture-induced cranial epidural abscess: case report and review of the literature. World Neurosurg. 2019 May;**125**:519-526

[77] Ullah W, Ahmad A, Mukhtar M, Virk HUH, Sarwar U, Figueredo V. Acupuncture-related cardiac complications: A systematic review. J Invasive Cardiol. 2019 Apr;**31**(4):E69-E72

[78] Corado SC, Graça Santos M, Quaresma L, Baltazar JR. Pneumothorax after acupuncture. BMJ Case Rep. 2019 Jun 11;12(6). pii: e228770.

[79] Ro A, Ponka JL. The hazard of iatrogenic pneumothorax in certain diagnostic and therapeutic procedures. Surg Gynecol Obstet. 1961 Jul;**113**:24-32

[80] Shafer N. Pneumothorax following "trigger point" injection. JAMA. 1970 Aug 17;**213**(7):1193

[81] Cheng J, Abdi S. Complications of joint, tendon and muscle injections. Tech Reg Anesth Pain Manag. 2007 Jul;**11**(3):141-147

[82] Usman F, Bajwa A, Shujaat A, Cury J. Retrosternal abscess after trigger point injections in a pregnant woman: a case report. J Med Case Rep. 2011 Aug 23;**5**:403

[83] Ahiskalioglu EO, Alici HA, Dostbil A, Celik M, Ahiskalioglu A, Aksoy M. Pneumothorax after trigger point injection: a case report and review of literature. J Back Musculoskelet Rehabil. 2016 Nov 21;**29**(4):895-897

[84] Soriano PK, Bhattarai M, Vogler CN, Hudali TH. A case of trigger point injection induced hypokalemic paralysis. Am J Case Rep. 2017 Apr 26;**18**:454-457

[85] Choe JY, Kim JK, Lee DE, Seo KS, Park JB, Lee MJ, et al. Descending necrotizing mediastinitis after a trigger point injection. Clin Exp Emerg Med. 2017 Sep 30;**4**(3):182-185

[86] Lee DG, Chang MC. Dorsal scapular nerve injury after trigger point injection into the rhomboid major muscle: a case

report. J Back Musculoskelet Rehabil. 2018 Feb 6;**31**(1):211-214

[87] De la Torre CG, Poluha RL, Lora VM. Araújo Oliveira Ferreira DM, Stuginski-Barbosa J, Bonjardim LR, Cury AADB, Conti PCR. Botulinum toxin type A applications for masticatory myofascial pain and trigeminal neuralgia: what is the evidence regarding adverse effects? Clin Oral Investig. 2019 Sep;**23**(9):3411-3421

[88] Camões-Barbosa A, Ribeiro IM, Medeiros L. Contralateral upper limb weakness following botulinum toxin A injection for poststroke spasticity. Acta Med Port. 2019 Apr;**26**:32(13)

[89] Mozafari N, Saffaei A, Alizadeh M, Shabani M. Cutaneous necrotic lesion: A wonderful delay adverse effect of interferon beta-1b injection for multiple sclerosis treatment. J Cosmet Dermatol. 2019 Aug;**22**

[90] Yürük D, Yılmaz A, Özgencil GE, Aşık İ. Acute rhabdomyolysis following epidural steroid injection: An unusual complication in a patient with low back pain. Agri. 2019 Jul;**31**(3):150-152

[91] Marcus F, Claude EV, Josephine M, Teyang A. An Exceptional cause of acute limb ischemia: Nicolau Syndrome-single-center experience with 4 Cases. Ann Vasc Surg. 2019 Jul;58:383.e7-383.e11.

[92] Kang HY, Kim JE, Kim YJ, Park SW, Kim Y. An unusual delayed onset of systemic toxicity after fluoroscopy-guided cervical epidural steroid injection with levobupivacaine: A case report. Pain Pract. 2019 Sep;**19**(7):762-766

[93] Park HB, Kam M, Gwark JY. Association of steroid injection with soft-tissue calcification in lateral epicondylitis. J Shoulder Elbow Surg. 2019 Feb;**28**(2):304-309

[94] Al-Omari AA, Aleshawi AJ, Marei OA, Younes HMB, Alawneh KZ, ALQuran E, Mohaidat ZM. Avascular necrosis of the femoral head after single steroid intra-articular injection. Eur J Orthop Surg Traumatol. 2020 Feb;**30**(2):193-197

[95] Lobaton GO, Marrache M, Petrusky O, Cohen DB, Jain A. Devastating vertebral osteomyelitis after epidural steroid injection: a case report. JBJS Case Connect. 2019 Dec;**9**(4):e0028

[96] Quincer E, Jaggi P. Nicolau Syndrome: A rare complication following intramuscular injection. J Pediatr. 2019 Sep;212:238-238.e2.

[97] Anderson SE, Lubberts B, Strong AD, Guss D, Johnson AH, DiGiovanni CW. Adverse events and their risk factors following intra-articular corticosteroid injections of the ankle or subtalar joint. Foot Ankle Int. 2019 Jun;**40**(6):622-628

[98] Kim BR, Lee JW, Lee E, Kang Y, Ahn JM, Kang HS. Intra-articular facet joint steroid injection-related adverse events encountered during 11,980 procedures. Eur Radiol. 2020 Mar;**30**(3):1507-1516

[99] Wang RN, Naraghi L. Oculomotor Nerve Palsy in the Emergency Department: A Complication of Epidural Injection. J Emerg Med. 2019 Nov 18. pii: S0736-4679(19)30841-8.

[100] Petrin Z, Marino RJ, Oleson CV, Simon JI, McCormick ZL. Paralysis following lumbar interlaminar epidural steroid injection in the absence of hematoma: A case of congestive myelopathy due to spinal dural arteriovenous fistula and a review of the literature. Am J Phys Med Rehabil. 2019 Oct;**7**

[101] Rensma HG, Van de Kerkhof-Van Bon B. Severe pain and skin

discolouration after injection: Nicolau syndrome, a rare complication. Ned Tijdschr Geneeskd. 2019 Oct 17;163. pii: D4001.

[102] Hu Y, Wang Y, Tong Y. Optic perineuritis secondary to hyaluronic acid injections: a case report. BMC Ophthalmol. 2019 Nov 27;**19**(1):241

[103] Lee JH, Wang SI, Noh SJ, Ham DH, Kim KB. Osteonecrosis of the medial tibial plateau after intra-articular corticosteroid injection: A case report. Medicine (Baltimore). 2019 Nov;**98**(44):e17248

[104] Ali D, El Khoumsi M, Gorur Y, Cardos B, Villalba NL. Rare case of ischaemic stroke following cervical transforaminal injection. Eur J Case Rep Intern Med. 2019 Mar 20;**6**(3):001082

[105] Rouientan A, Alizadeh Otaghvar H, Mahmoudvand H, Tizmaghz A. Rare complication of botox injection: a case report. World J Plast Surg. 2019 Jan;**8**(1):116-119

[106] Jani P, Morley HL, Shetty N. Iatrogenic adrenal suppression following caudal epidural and facet joint injection. BMJ Case Rep. 2019 Feb 21;12(2). pii: e225828.

[107] Desai K, Warade AC, Jha AK, Pattankar S. Injection-related iatrogenic peripheral nerve injuries: Surgical experience of 354 operated cases. Neurol India. 2019 Jan-Feb;67(Supplement):S82-S91.

[108] Park CW, Cho WC, Son BC. Iatrogenic injury to the sciatic nerve due to intramuscular injection: A Case Report. Korean J Neurotrauma. 2019 Apr 8;**15**(1):61-66

[109] Ali SS, Shaw AE, Oselkin M, Bragin I. Iatrogenic spinal epidural hematoma associated with intracranial hypotension. Cureus. 2019 Mar 4;**11**(3):e4171

[110] Sencan S, Cüce İ, Gündüz OH. Use of fluoroscopic-guided transsacral block for the treatment of iatrogenic post-injection sciatic neuropathy: Report of three cases. Turk J Phys Med Rehabil. 2019 Nov 22;**65**(4):406-410

[111] Lee JH, Lee H, Jo DJ. An acute cervical epidural hematoma as a complication of dry needling. Spine (Phila Pa 1976). 2011 Jun;**36**(13):E891-E893

[112] McCutcheon L, Yelland MJ. Iatrogenic pneumothorax: Safety concerns when using acupuncture or dry needling in the thoracic region. Physical Therapy Reviews 16(2): 126-132. April 2011

[113] Brady S, McEvoy J, Dommerholt J, Doody C. Adverse events following trigger point dry needling: a prospective survey of chartered physiotherapists. J Man Manip Ther. 2014 Aug;**22**(3):134-140

[114] Halle JS, Halle RJ. Pertinent dry needling considerations for minimizing adverse effects - Part one. Int J Sports Phys Ther. 2016 Aug;**11**(4):651-662

[115] Halle JS, Halle RJ. Pertinent dry needling considerations for minimizing adverse effects - Part two. Int J Sports Phys Ther. 2016 Oct;**11**(5):810-819

[116] McManus R, Cleary M. Radial nerve injury following dry needling. BMJ Case Rep. 2018 Jan 26;2018. pii: bcr-2017-221302.

[117] Berrigan WA, Whitehair CL, Zorowitz RD. Acute spinal epidural hematoma as a complication of dry needling: A case report. PM R. 2019 Mar;**11**(3):313-316

[118] Uzar T, Turkmen I, Menekse EB, Dirican A, Ekaterina P, Ozkaya S. A case with iatrogenic pneumothorax due to deep dry needling. Radiol Case Rep. 2018 Sep 20;**13**(6):1246-1248

[119] Kim DC, Glenzer S, Johnson A, Nimityongskul P. Deep infection following dry needling in a young athlete: an underreported complication of an increasingly prevalent modality: a case report. J Bone Joint Surg Am. 2018 Jul-Sep;**8**(3):e73

[120] McDowell JM, Kohu SH, Betts D. Safe acupuncture and dry needling during pregnancy: New Zealand physiotherapists' opinion and practice. Journal of Integrative Medicine. January 2019;**17**(1):30-37

[121] Leung JS. Complementary medicine, acupuncture, and pneumothorax. Hong Kong Med J. 2002;**8**:225

[122] Park KY, Jang WS, Kim IS, Ko EJ, Seo SJ. Hong CK Multiple epidermal cysts as a complication of gold acupuncture. Ann Dermatol. 2014 Jun;**26**(3):405-406

[123] Bashey S, Lee DS, Kim G. Extensive facial sclerosing lipogranulomatosis as a complication of cosmetic acupuncture. Dermatol Surg. 2015 Apr;**41**(4):513-516

[124] Henneghien C, Bruart J, Remacle P. A new iatrogenic pathology: pneumothorax after acupuncture. Rev Pneumol Clin. 1984;**40**(3):197-199

[125] Cantan R, Milesi-Defrance N, Hardenberg K, Vernet M, Messant I, Freysz M. Bilateral pneumothorax and tamponade after acupuncture. Presse Med. 2003 Feb 22;**32**(7):311-312

[126] Morrone N, Freire JA, Ferreira AK, Dourado AM. Iatrogenic pneumothorax caused by acupuncture. Rev Paul Med. 1990 Jul-Aug;**108**(4):189-191

[127] Marchuk IK, Kuz'mich VN, Marchuk LI, Ordynskiĭ NL. Iatrogenic pneumothorax. Lik Sprava. 1993 Oct-Dec;(10-12):81-82.

[128] De Groot M. Acupuncture complications, contraindications and informed consent. Forsch Komplementarmed Klass Naturheilkd. 2001 Oct;**8**(5):256-262

[129] Ronconi G, De Giorgio F, Ricci E, Maggi L, Spagnolo AG, Ferrara PE. Pneumothorax following dry needling treatment: legal and ethical aspects. Ig Sanita Pubbl. 2016 Sep-Oct;**72**(5):505-512

[130] Steentjes K, de Vries LM, Ridwan BU, Wijgman AJ. Infection of a hip prosthesis after dry needling. Ned Tijdschr Geneeskd. 2016;**160**:A9364

[131] Valgardsson AS, Gudbjartsson T. Bilateral pneumothoraces in a pregnant woman following acupuncture – a case report. Laeknabladid. 2019 Jan;**105**(1):19-21

[132] Zhao DY, Zhang GL. Clinical analysis on 38 cases of pneumothorax induced by acupuncture or acupoint injection. Zhongguo Zhen Jiu. 2009 Mar;**29**(3):239-242

[133] Larsson AS, Jørgensen IM. Acupuncture-induced bilateral pneumothorax in a 16-year-old boy. Ugeskr Laeger. 2018 Feb 26;180(9). pii: V10170804.

[134] Murray PI, Aboteen N. Complication of acupuncture in a patient with Behçet's disease. Br J Ophthalmol. 2002 Apr;**86**(4):476-477

[135] Cummings M, Ross-Marrs R, Gerwin R. Pneumothorax complication of deep dry needling demonstration. Acupunct Med. 2014 Dec;**32**(6):517-519

[136] Patrick BS. Acupuncture complication--a case report. J Miss State Med Assoc. 2005 Jul;**46**(7):195-197

Chapter 2

Difficult Intravenous Access and Its Management

Handan Eren

Abstract

Difficult intravenous access (DIVA) may occur due to several factors, such as the demographic and clinical characteristics of the patients (age, sex, height, weight, ethnicity, IV drugs history, and medical history), health professional's experience, device characteristics, site of insertion, and vein characteristics. Difficult intravenous access leads to repeated insertion attempts that might prove to be uncomfortable for the patients, frustrating and challenging for the health professionals, and expensive for the health institutions. The practitioners must develop the awareness of the factors capable of increasing the difficulty of defining the appropriate vein for cannulation through their varied experiences with vein location and vascular access.

Keywords: difficult cannulation, patient, practitioner

1. Introduction

Difficult intravenous access (DIVA) is defined as a catheter insertion condition when the catheter cannot be entered into the vein in one attempt [1]. A published systematic review and meta-analyses reported a failure rate of up to 30% on the first attempt of peripheral intravenous cannulation [2]. Other research identifies a failure rate ranging from 10%–40%, which is consistent with the findings from a study by Witting (2012), who reported that 39% of first time attempts at peripheral intravenous cannulation (PIVC) failed [3, 4].

DIVA may occur due to several factors and lead to multiple repetitive attempts to gain peripheral venous access, which causes the patients to experience pain and anxiety and the healthcare professionals to feel inadequate [1]. In addition, as the number of materials used in the repetitive attempts increases and the treatment plan for the patient is delayed, the patient care costs also increase [5, 6]. Therefore, it is crucial for healthcare professionals to be aware of the factors that may lead to this condition, including several negativities, to understand how to manage it [7, 8]. The guidelines available for peripheral intravenous insertion mainly focus on site selection and insertion, and there is a lack of established guidelines on how to recognize or manage DIVA [1, 9–11]. In this context, the present study was aimed to provide basic information regarding the risk factors for difficult peripheral intravenous cannulation and its management.

IntechOpen

2. Individual factors

The individual risk factors associated with DIVA are age, gender, ethnicity, body mass index, health status, medical history, and vein characteristics of the patients [7, 12–14].

2.1 Age

The age of the individual might affect the intravenous catheter insertion. With increasing age, the vein diameter expands, thereby increasing the visibility and palpability of the veins [13, 15]. Therefore, it could be relatively difficult to determine the appropriate vein in neonates and children. According to the literature, the success rate of catheter insertion in the first attempt observed in the pediatric clinics varies between 44% and 86% [15, 16]. However, similar rates are observed in older ages. This might be because of the decreased elasticity of the blood vessels at an advanced age, which could contribute to DIVA. In the studies conducted by Van Loon et al. with 3586 participants and by Armenteros-Yeguas et al. (2017) with 135 participants, no relationship between the age of the individuals and DIVA was observed, although DIVA was observed to be related to the presence of chronic disease and medical treatment. The increased possibility of chronic diseases in advanced age would result in a medical treatment history, leading to DIVA [12, 13].

2.2 Gender

Studies have reported that gender is a risk factor for difficult venous access. Jacobson and Winslow (2005) reported that catheter insertion procedure is more difficult in women compared to men. This could be explained by the smaller caliber of peripheral veins in women [17]. Piredda et al. (2019) also reported gender as one of the risk factors for difficult venous access and that the procedure could be relatively difficult in women. In the same study, 99.4% of the women who underwent lymph node dissection experienced DIVA, suggesting an association; the multivariate analysis conducted in the study revealed that lymph node dissection did not exert a statistically significant effect on difficult cannulation [7].

2.3 Ethnicity

Individuals with different ethnicities may have different skin colors, and peripheral intravenous cannulation (PIVC) might be difficult in certain individuals of particular skin color. A narrative review published in 2010 by Sabri et al. reported an association between skin color and DIVA [18]. Jacobson and Winslow (2005) also reported that catheter insertion was more difficult in individuals with dark and/or tough skins [17].

2.4 Body mass index

Body mass index (BMI) is a measure of body fat based on the height and weight of the individual. An increase in weight may cause an increase in the adipose tissue and, therefore, a decrease in the visibility of the veins, rendering the catheter insertion difficult [14, 17]. Several studies have reported body mass index as a risk factor for difficult catheter insertion [7, 13, 14]. Sebbane et al. (2013) reported that underweight patients (BMI < 18.5 kg/m2) face a higher risk of DIVA. They stated that this result may be related to vein mobility [19]. However, Lapostolle et al. (2007) found no association with BMI and IV failure [20]. Fields et al. (2014) also did not find an association between obesity and DIVA [21]. This results may be related to patients characteristic.

2.5 Patient's health conditions

It is reported that the physiological and psychological conditions of the individuals exert an effect on their venous structure [12, 14]. It is elucidated that certain chronic diseases may cause the deterioration and hardening of the vascular structure, rendering the catheter placement process difficult. Cancer, diabetes mellitus, and vascular diseases are among the conditions that render vein access difficult [7, 13, 14]. Intravenous chemotherapy treatment or surgical procedure/dissection of the lymph nodes associated with breast cancer reduces the visibility and palpability of the veins. Furthermore, circulation problems, which are among the advanced complications of diabetes mellitus, and conditions such as coronary artery disease and the associated medical treatments, may directly cause the deterioration of the vein structure [7, 8, 12, 17]. Loon et al. (2019) reported that diabetes mellitus and chemotherapy treatment were associated with forced catheter intervention [13]. Piredda and colleagues (2019), as well as Carr and colleagues (2016), stated that the treatments of diabetes, venous disease, and cancer are closely associated with the difficult catheter intervention as they cause the reduction of blood vessel diameter [7, 17].

Dehydration is another risk factor for difficult catheter insertion as it causes the blood volume to decrease and the venous pressure to decrease, thereby rendering the detection of veins and consequently catheter insertion difficult. Dehydration is reported to lead to repeated catheter interventions [22]. However, in the study conducted by Sharp et al. (2018), a decrease of 0.57 mm in the diameter of the median cubital vein and 0.33 mm in the diameter of the cephalic vein was observed after oral rehydration. This could be related to the fact that drinking water may stimulate the sympathetic nervous system, which would then decrease the vessel diameter [23].

Emotional conditions of the individuals may also affect catheter intervention. Anxiety may lead to peripheral vasoconstriction, thereby increasing the difficulty of cannulation [24]. Having the patient lie in the during catheterization, using the muscle tensing technique, informing the patient regarding the procedure, and gaining the patient's confidence are a few factors that may reduce anxiety in the patients prior to the procedure, enabling better cannulation [25].

2.6 Patient's medical history

Medical histories of the individuals, particularly the previous history of difficulty with punctures or insertion of catheters, may be the risk factors for DIVA due to their effect on the vascular structure [13, 14]. Intravenous chemotherapy treatment is one of the most serious causes of the disruption of the vascular structure. Chemotherapy drugs (vesicants, irritants) cause complications such as phlebitis, infiltration, extravasation, thrombophlebitis, and septicemia, manifesting as pain, redness, ulceration, and necrosis along the vein, and stimulate the sympathetic nervous system, thereby causing the vessels to contract and decreasing their fullness and visibility [26]. Similarly, fluids with high osmolarity, the blood, and the blood products may damage the vascular endothelium. Repeated attempts of these treatments may be a risk factor for DIVA [27].

2.7 Vein characteristics

The vascular structure may differ from individual to individual. The diameter, visibility, palpability, and superficiality (or depth) of the vein are important factors to be considered when determining the appropriate vein for PIVC [8]. A vein with a wide diameter is easily visible and palpable. Van Loon et al. reported that non-palpable invisible veins and the veins less than 3 mm in diameter after tourniquet application lead to DIVA [13]. Jacobson and Winslow (2005) reported that failed IV insertions were associated with higher degrees of difficulty arising from vein a variable, such as vein rolled or vein was resistant to puncture.

3. Factors related to health professionals

It is reported that difficult peripheral intravenous cannulation affects 10%–24% of all hospitalized adults and is associated with higher rates of catheter failure. This situation may lead to several complications, such as phlebitis, extravasation, hemorrhage, catheter-related infection, and sepsis [6, 18]. In order to prevent these complications, healthcare professionals must be aware of the risk factors for DIVA. The practitioners' knowledge and skill regarding catheter insertion and their clinical experience are the health professional-related factors for difficult cannulation [7, 14]. The literature states that the experience of the practitioner with catheter insertion is associated with forced catheter intervention. Rippey et al. (2016) reported that the practitioner's experience influenced the success of catheter placement in a single attempt [28]. Van Loon et al. (2019) reported that the prediction that the practitioner might have a difficult catheter intervention was associated with DIVA [13]. Rodriguez-Calero et al. (2020) reported no relationship between the clinical experience of the practitioners and DIVA and stated that catheter insertion could only be associated with the patients and their treatment [14].

The success of vascular access and conducting the procedure in a short duration are important for patient safety and satisfaction. Determining the appropriate vein, using the appropriate materials, and placing the catheter with the right technique would make the procedure convenient for both patient and the healthcare professional. Therefore, the practitioners must possess adequate knowledge and skills of cannulation [29, 30].

4. Management of difficult venous access

PIVC is expected to be performed in a single attempt. In the cases where the catheter cannot be inserted in a single attempt, it is recommended to limit the number of insertions by a single practitioner to two [29]. However, this is not possible in certain cases. Therefore, determining the appropriate vein and the appropriate catheter and using the most appropriate technique to access the vein is important for the prevention and control of DIVA caused due to factors related to either the patient or the practitioner [8, 11, 14, 18].

4.1 Assessment of the appropriate vein in difficult venous access

Determining the appropriate vein prior to catheter insertion is important for performing the procedure conveniently. Plump veins are distinctly visible and palpable, and therefore, easier to detect. In order to determine if the catheter insertion procedure would be challenging, the veins should be graded. Certain vein grading scales have been developed for application in adults and pediatric patients [13, 31, 32]. The Adult Difficult IntraVenous Access (A-DIVA) scale developed and updated by Van Loon et al. (2019) includes a known history of difficult intravenous access, an expectation of difficult intravenous access by the practitioner prior to the intravenous cannulation, the inability to detect a dilated vein through palpation and/or visualization of the extremity, and a target vein diameter of less than 3 mm. A higher score on the A-DIVA scale indicates a higher risk of difficult intravenous access [13] (**Table 1**). In the vein grading scale developed by Lenhardt et al. (2002) the following factors were included: 1) The veins are completely invisible and not palpable; 2) The veins are visible although not palpable; 3) The veins are hardly visible although palpable, 4: The veins are visible and palpable; 5) The veins are distinctly visible and palpable. This scale may be used to evaluate the veins, although access to the veins rated 1 on this scale could be rather difficult [32].

Vein grading/assessment scales for small patient groups are different. The Difficult IntraVenous Access (DIVA) scale developed by Yen et al. (2008) included the visibility and palpability of the vein, and the age, skin color, and premature status of the patients as evaluation parameters. The obtained scores ranged from 0 to 11. If the obtained score was four or higher, it indicated difficult vascular access with a 50% probability of failure [31]. The scale was reviewed by Riker et al. (2011) who reduced the parameters to only 3, namely visibility of vein, palpability of vein, and age of the patient. The scale has also been adapted to the Turkish population by removing the parameter of skin color. The prediction of whether the procedure would be difficult prior to the PIVC is crucial as it prevents possible complications (**Table 2**) [31, 33]. Therefore, it is recommended that healthcare professionals use these scales [29].

The more visible and more palpable the vein preferred for PIVC, the more convenient the procedure would be. Dorsal metacarpal veins, basilica, and cephalic veins are the frequently preferred ones for PIVC. In particular, for ongoing intravenous treatments, the IV entry site should be located distal to the arm, and each attempt should be further proximal compared to the next attempt. Leg and foot veins should be avoided as much as possible due to the risk of lower extremity embolism involved [34]. However, this order of vein preference may change in the cases where veins are not easily visible and palpable. If there is a possibility of difficult cannulation, the upper arm basilica vein should be preferred because of its larger diameter. However, since this vein might be deep-seated, its visibility could be low; in which case; the procedure should be performed using palpation or vein imaging systems [35].

Another frequently preferred vein to avoid difficult venous access is the antecubital vein. The large diameter and the superficial location of this vein render it easily visible or palpable. However, with this vein, catheter stabilization could be difficult as this vein is located in the elbow joint [34]. Panebianco et al. (2009) reported that, with an increase in the diameter of the veins (92% success at 0.6 cm)

Factor	Score
Is there a known history of a difficult intravenous access?	1
Do you expect a failed first attempt or a difficult intravenous access?	1
Is there an inability to identify a dilated vein by palpating the upper extremity?	1
Is there an inability to identify a dilated vein by visualizing the upper extremity?	1
Has the largest dilated vein a diameter less than 3 millimeters?	1

Table 1.
The additive A-DIVA scale [13].

Predictor variable	Score		
Visibility	Visible = 0		Not visible = 2
Palpability	Palpable = 0		Not palpable = 2
Age	≥36 months = 0	12–35 months = 1	<12 months = 3
Prematurity	Not premature = 0		Premature = 3
Skin shade	Light = 0	Dark = 1	

Table 2.
DIVA score [33].

and within the vein depth range of 1.2 to 1.4 cm, the success of catheter placement increases. An ultrasound device should be used to determine the diameter and the depth of the veins [36].

4.1.1 Techniques to increase vein visibility in difficult venous access

The literature recommends the use of ultrasound and vein imaging devices for the detection of veins with low visibility and palpability. Information regarding the diameter and the depth of the veins may be obtained using the ultrasound technique. Previous studies have demonstrated that the use of an ultrasound device increased the rate of successful catheter placement at the first attempt, particularly in difficult venous access [16, 37]. Moreover, it is reported that the use of vascular imaging devices, which enables the visualization of the veins using infrared rays, prior to the procedure is particularly effective in pediatric patients and the individuals with impaired vascular structure receiving intravenous chemotherapy treatment (**Figure 1**) [1, 18, 30]. Eren (2018) reported that the use of a vein imaging device in patients with difficult venous access significantly shortened the time to determine the appropriate vein compared to the use of a tourniquet and fist-clenching techniques [30]. In a study carried out by Caglar et al. (2019) with preterm infants, it is found that success of the first attempt was significantly higher in the infrared and transilluminator groups than in the control group ($p \leq .05$). It is also found that time to successful cannulation was significantly lower for the infrared group (8.70 ± 2.56 seconds) than for the transilluminator group (45.27 ± 30.83 seconds) and the control group [38]. Considering the patient outcomes of studies conducted using the ultrasound device, ultrasound guidance increases the likelihood of successful peripheral cannulation in difficult access patients. Ultrasound guided peripheral IV catheter placement has a greater success rate with fewer skin punctures, decreased time for IV catheter placement, and fewer complications [39, 40]. Chiriloco et al. (2015) reported that first attempt success was 85% with using ultrasound at 200 patients with DIVA. They also said that patient satisfaction was higher in ultrasound guided vascular access group than traditional peripheral venous catheter insertion group [41]. In summary, ultrasound guided insertion significantly improved first attempt success rates and demonstrated higher patient satisfaction scores when compared to conventional venous catheter use.

Besides these techniques, tourniquet application, hot application, topical vasodilator application, fist-clenching, holding the arm below the chest level, hitting the vein, and massaging may be used to make the veins fuller for easier vein determination [30, 32, 34, 38, 42–44]. Tourniquet application is one of the most commonly used techniques for vein determination. The literature recommends the use of a sphygmomanometer rather than a tourniquet for the individuals with sensitive/fragile veins and those with a risk of difficult venous access. It is suggested to inflate

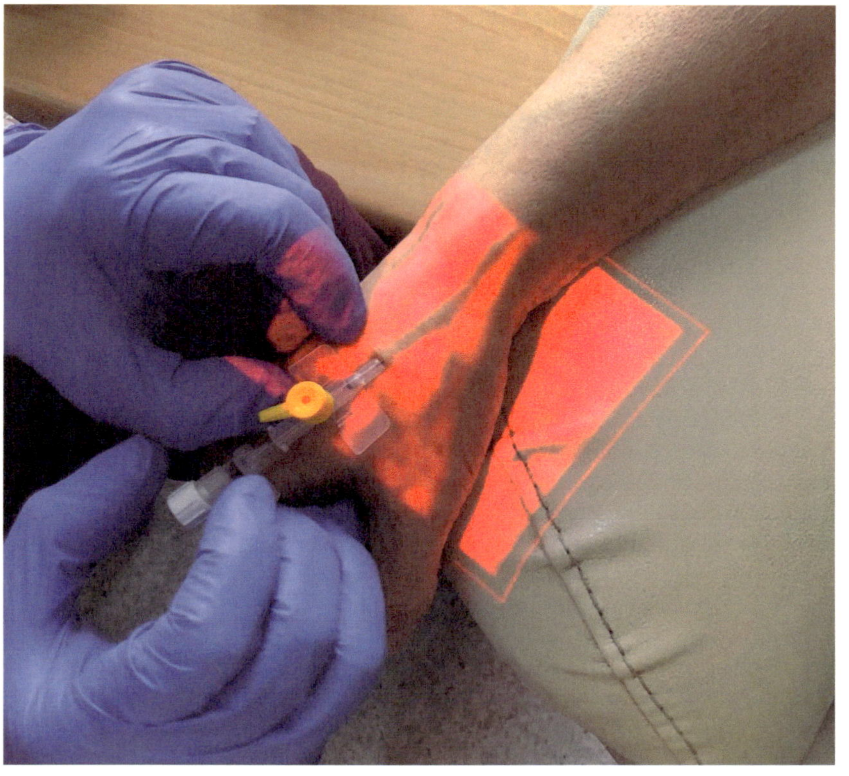

Figure 1.
PIVC used with vein imaging device.

the manometer to the level of the individual's diastolic blood pressure [38, 43]. Nitroglycerin, a topical vasodilator, increases the visibility of the vein, although it may not be suitable for every patient as it is absorbed into the skin [45]. Another technique, named hot application, assists in expanding the veins to make them fuller. Studies have demonstrated that hot application facilitates vein detection and catheter insertion in patients with DIVA [43, 46].

4.2 Determination of the appropriate catheter and vein entry angle in difficult venous access

The size of intravenous catheters [14, 15, 18, 21, 23, 25] is referred to as the gauge. The diameter and the length of the cannula vary with the size of the catheter. As the number/size of the catheter increases, the cannula diameter decreases. In addition, different lengths are available for the catheters of the same size [29, 34]. Generally, a 20-gauge to a 24-gauge catheter is preferred for peripheral catheterization. Peripheral catheters larger than 20 gauge in size are more likely to cause phlebitis. A 22 to 24 gauge catheter for neonates, pediatric patients, and older adults generally minimizes the insertion-related trauma. A 20-gauge to 24-gauge catheter should be used based on the vein size for blood transfusion; when rapid transfusion is required, a larger-size catheter gauge is recommended [29].

The catheter should be placed at an angle of 10–30 degrees to the skin, and after entering the vein at the PIVC, the angle should be reduced. However, the veins that are superficial, thin, slippery, and present a risk of difficult venous access should be entered at an angle of 30–45 degrees to the skin, from the lower side of the entry point and parallel to the vein, and immediately after entering the vein, the angle should be reduced to 15 degrees [34]. In the process of catheter placement with the assistance of the ultrasound technique, if a vessel is 16 mm deep and is entered at a 45° angle to the vein, then a catheter with a minimum length of 23 mm is required to reach the vessel. At a 30° angle, the catheter would have to be 32 mm to reach the anterior wall of the vessel [36].

5. Conclusion

Difficult venous access is characterized by non-visible and non-palpable veins and is caused by the various patient- and practitioner-related factors, such as age, obesity, history of chemotherapy, and vein characteristics of the patients, and the clinical experience of the practitioners [1, 7, 8, 12]. Understanding these factors for DIVA may facilitate the management of difficult venous access and improve patient outcomes in this population. In difficult intravenous catheter intervention, determining the appropriate vein and placing the catheter with the appropriate technique is required. Evaluation of veins before catheter insertion is crucial in determining the appropriate vein. For this, vein grading scales should be used [31, 32, 47]. Techniques to increase vein fullness (e.g. fist clenching, hot application, topical vasodilator, tapping) can be used to determine the vein, or ultrasound and vein imaging devices can be used to view veins [2, 23, 30, 35, 43, 46]. In addition, difficult venous access guidelines, which are limited in the literature, need to be developed.

Author details

Handan Eren
Department of Nursing, Yalova University, Yalova, Turkey

*Address all correspondence to: erennhandan@gmail.com

References

[1] Sou V, McManus C, Mifflin N, Frost SA, Ale J, Alexandrou EA. Clinical pathway for the management of difficult venous access. BMC Nursing. 2017;16:1-7.

[2] Van Loon FHJ, Buise MP, Claassen JJF, Dierick-van Daele ATM, Bouwman ARA. Comparison of ultrasound guidance with palpation and direct visualization for peripheral vein cannulation in adult patients: A systematic review and meta-analysis. British Journal Anaesthesia. 2018;121:358-366.

[3] Witting MD. IV access difficulty: Incidence and delays in an urban emergency department. Journal of Emergency Medicine. 2012;42(4):483-487.

[4] Leidel BA, Kirchhoff C, Bogner V, Stegmaier J, Mutschler W, Kanz KG, Braunstein, V. Is the intraosseous access route fast and efficacious compared to conventional central venous catheterization in adult patients under resuscitation in the emergency department? A prospective observational pilot study. Patient Safety in Surgery. 2009; 3(1):24.

[5] Scoppettuolo G, Pittiruti M, Pitoni S, Dolcetti L, Emoli A, Mitidieri A, Migliorini I, Annetta M.G. Ultrasound-guided "short" midline catheters for difficult venous access in the emergency department: A retrospective analysis. International Journal Emergency Medicine. 2016;9(3):1-7.

[6] Miliani K, Taravella R, Thillard D, Chauvin V, Martin E, Edouard S, Astagneau P. Peripheral venous catheter-related adverse events: Evaluation from a multicentre epidemiological study in France. PLoS ONE. 2017;12:1-17.

[7] Piredda M, Fiorini J, Facchinetti G, Biagioli V, Marchetti A, Conti F, Iacorossi L, Giannarelli D, Matarese M, De Marinis MG. Risk factors for a difficult intravenous access: A multicentre study comparing nurses' beliefs to evidence. Journal of Clinical Nursing. 2019;28:3492-3504.

[8] Engström Å, Forsberg A. Peripheral intravenous catheter difficulty–A clinical survey of registered nurse and critical care nurse performance. Journal of Clinical Nursing. 2019;28(3-4):686-694.

[9] Abolfotouh M A, Salam M, Ala'a Bani-Mustafa DW, Balkhy HH. Prospective study of incidence and predictors of peripheral intravenous catheter-induced complications. Therapeutics and clinical risk management. 2014;10:993-1001.

[10] Keogh S, Shelverton C, Flynn J, Mihala G, Mathew S, Davies KM, Marsh N, Rickard C M. Implementation and evaluation of short peripheral intravenous catheter flushing guidelines: a stepped wedge cluster randomised trial. BMC medicine 2020;18(1):1-11.

[11] Ho KH, Cheung DS. (2012). Guidelines on timing in replacing peripheral intravenous catheters. Journal of Clinical Nursing. 2012;21(11-12):1499-1506.

[12] Armenteros-Yeguas V, Gárate-Echenique L, Tomás-López MA, Cristóbal-Domínguez E, Moreno-de Gusmão B, Miranda-Serrano E, Moraza-Dulanto MI. Prevalence of difficult venous access and associated risk factors in highly complex hospitalised patients. Journal of Clinical Nursing. 2017;26(23-24):4267-4275.

[13] Van Loon FH, Van Hooff LW, de Boer HD, Koopman SS, Buise MP,

Korsten HH, Bouwman AR. The modified A-DIVA scale as a predictive tool for prospective identification of adult patients at risk of a difficult intravenous access: A multicenter validation study. Journal of Clinical Medicine. 2019;8(2):144-156.

[14] Rodríguez-Calero M A., Blanco-Mavillard I, Morales-Asencio JM, Fernández-FernándezI,Castro-SánchezE, de Pedro-Gómez J E. Defining risk factors associated with difficult peripheral venous cannulation: A systematic review and meta-analysis. Heart & Lung. 2020;49(3):273-286.

[15] Carr PJ, Rippey JC, Budgeon CA, Cooke ML, Higgins N, Rickard CM. Insertion of peripheral intravenous cannulae in the Emergency Department: factors associated with first-time insertion success. Journal of Vascular Access. 2016;17(2):182-90.

[16] Lininger R. Pediatric peripheral i.v. insertion success rates. Journal of Pediatric Nursing 2003; 29(5) 351-4.

[17] Jacobson AF, Winslow EH. Variables influencing intravenous catheter insertion difficulty and failure: An analysis of 339 intravenous catheter insertions. Heart and Lung: The Journal of Acute and Critical Care. 2005;34:345-359.

[18] Sabri, A., Szalas, J., Holmes, K. S., Labib, L., Mussivand, T. Failed attempts and improvement strategies in peripheral intravenous catheterization. Bio-medical materials and engineering. 2013;23(1-2):93-108.

[19] Sebbane M, Claret PG, Lefebvre S, Mercier G, Rubenovitch J, Jreige R, Eledjam JJ, de La Coussaye JE. Predicting peripheral venous access difficulty in the emergency department using body mass index and a clinical evaluation of venous accessibility. The Journal of emergency medicine. 2013;44(2): 299-305.

[20] Lapostolle F, Catineau J, Garrigue B, Monmrteau V, Houssaye T, Vecci I, Hospital B, Crocheton N, Adnet F. Prospective evaluation of peripheral venous access difficulty in emergency care. Intensive Care Med. 2007;33(8):1452-1457.

[21] Fields JM, Piela NE, Au AK, Ku BS. Risk factors associated with difficult venous access in adult ED patients. The American journal of emergency medicine. 2014;32(10):1179-1182.

[22] Diaconu CI, Fox RJ, Grattan A, Rae-Grant A, Lu M, Gornik HL, Kim SH. Hydration status substantially affects chronic cerebrospinal venous insufficiency assessments. Neurology: Clinical Practice. 2013;3(5):386-91.

[23] Sharp R, Childs J, Bulmer AC, Esterman A. The effect of oral hydration and localised heat on peripheral vein diameter and depth: A randomised controlled trial. Applied Nursing Research. 2018;42:83-88.

[24] Dougherty L, Lister S. The Royal Marsden Manual of Clinical Nursing Procedures, 9th ed. John Wiley & Sons, Hoboken, NJ; 2015. 148 p.

[25] McIntyre-Patton L, Wanderski S, Graef D, Woessner L, Baker R. Randomized trial evaluating the effectiveness of a leg crossing and muscle tensing technique on decreasing vasovagal symptoms among pediatric and young adult patients undergoing peripheral IV catheter insertion. Journal of Pediatric Nursing. 2018;38:53-56.

[26] Özkaraman A, Yeşilbakan OU. Periferal intravenöz kemoterapi uygulamasına yönelik hemşirelik yönetimi. Osmangazi Journal of Medicine.2015;36(1):27-34.

[27] Doellman D, Hadaway L, BoweGeddes LA, Franklin M, LeDonne J, Papke O'Donnell L, Pettit J,

Schulmeister L, Stranz MP. Infiltration and extravasation. The Art and Science of Infusion Nursing. 2009;32:203-211.

[28] Rippey JC, Carr PJ, Cooke M, Higgins N, Rickard CM. Predicting and preventing peripheral intravenous cannula insertion failure in the emergency department: Clinician 'gestalt'wins again. Emergency Medicine Australasia. 2016;28(6):658-665.

[29] Gorski L, Hadaway L, Hagle ME, McGoldrick M, Orr M, Doellman D. Infusion Therapy Standards of Practice. Journal of Infusion Nursing. 2016;39(1S): 1-169.

[30] Eren H. The effect of the vascular imaging device and fist clenching method on vein visibility in patients who are receiving chemotherapy [thesis]. Ankara: Gazi University, 2018.

[31] Gerçeker GÖ, Gümüş M, Yardimci F, Polat ME, Eroğlu B, İslamoğlu A. Psychometric Properties of The Turkish Version of The Difficult Intravenous Access Score for Children. Dokuz Eylül Üniversitesi Hemşirelik Fakültesi Elektronik Dergisi. 2017; 10(3) 153-158.

[32] Lenhardt R, Seybold T, Kimberger O, Stoiser B, Sessler DI. Local Warming and Insertion of Peripheral Venous Cannulas: Single Blinded Prospective Randomised Controlled Trial and Single Blinded Randomised Crossover Trial. British Medical Journal. 2002;325:409-503.

[33] Riker MW, Kennedy C, W Infrey BS, Yen K, Dowd MD. Validation and refinement of the difficult intravenous access score: a clinical prediction rule for identifying children with difficult intravenous access. Academic Emergency Medicine. 2011; 18(11):1129-34.

[34] Uzun Ş. İntravenöz sıvı tedavisi. In: Atabek-Aştı T, Karadağ A, editors. Hemşirelik esasları: Hemşirelik bilimi ve sanatı içinde. 2nd ed. İstanbul: Akademi Basın ve Yayıncılık; 2019. p. 699-730.

[35] Meyer P, Cronier P, Rousseau H, Vicaut E, Choukroun G, Chergui K, Maury E. Difficult peripheral venous access: clinical evaluation of a catheter inserted with the Seldinger method under ultrasound guidance. Journal of critical care. 2014;29(5):823-827.

[36] Panebianco NL, Fredette JM, Szyld D, Sagalyn EB, Pines JM, Dean AJ. What you see (sonographically) is what you get: vein and patient characteristics associated with successful ultrasound-guided peripheral intravenous placement in patients with difficult access. Academic Emergency Medicine. 2009;16(12):1298-1303.

[37] Gottlieb M, Sundaram T, Holladay D, Nakitende D. Ultrasound-guided peripheral intravenous line placement: a narrative review of evidence-based best practices. Western Journal of Emerg ency Medicine. 2017;18(6):1047.

[38] Caglar S, Büyükyilmaz F, Bakoglu I, Inal S, Salihoglu Ö. Efficacy of vein visualization devices for peripheral intravenous catheter placement in preterm infants: a randomized clinical trial. J. Perinat. Neonatal Nurs. 2019;33(1),:61-67.

[39] Doniger SJ, Ishimine P, Fox JC, Kanegaye JT. Randomized controlled trial of ultrasound-guided peripheral intravenous catheter placement versus traditional techniques in difficult-access pediatric patients. Pediatric emergency care. 2009;25(3):154-159.

[40] Chiricolo G, Balk A, Raio C, Wen W, Mihailos A, Ayala S. Higher success rates and satisfaction in difficult venous access patients with a guide wire–associated peripheral venous catheter. The American journal of emergency medicine. 2015;33(12):1742-1744.

[41] Yamagami Y, Tomita K, Tsujimoto T, Inoue T. Tourniquet application after local forearm warming to improve venodilation for peripheral intravenous cannulation in young and middle-aged adults: A single-blind prospective randomized controlled trial. International Journal of Nursing Studies. 2017;72:1-7.

[42] Egan G, Healy D, O'Neill H, Clarke-Moloney M, Grace PA, Walsh SR. Ultrasound guidance for difficult peripheral venous access: systematic review and meta-analysis. Emergency Medicine Journal. 2013;30(7):521-526.

[43] Bıyık Bayram Ş, Çalışkan N. Effects of local heat application before intravenous catheter insertion in chemotherapy patients. Journal of Clinical Nursing. 2016;25(11-12):1740-1747.

[44] Cantor-Peled G, Halak M, Ovadia-Blechman Z. Peripheral vein locating techniques. Imaging in Medicine. 2016;8(3):83-88.

[45] Shrestha N, Acharya U, Shrestha PS, Acharya SP, Karki B, Dhakal SS. Topical nitroglycerin for management of peripheral extravasation of vasopressors: a case report. Oxford Medical Case Reports. 2020;(8):omaa066.

[46] Korkut S, Karadağ S, Doğan Z. The Effectiveness of Local Hot and Cold Applications on Peripheral Intravenous Catheterization: A Randomized Controlled Trial. Journal of PeriAnesthesia Nursing. 2020; 35(6):597-602.

[47] Yen K, Riegert A, Gorelick MH. Derivation of the ZIVG score: a clinical prediction rule for the identification of children with difficult intravenous access.Pediatric Emergency Care. 2008;24(3):143-7.

Chapter 3

Self-Management of Blood Pressure Control at Home in Chronic Kidney Disease: Nursing Interventions and Health Gains

Dilar Costa and Filipa Aguiar

Abstract

One of the advantages of HBPM (Home Blood Pressure Measurement) compared to office measurement is being a strong predictor of cardiovascular morbidity and mortality in hypertensive patients, including those with chronic kidney disease (CKD). However, studies with renal patients not dependent on dialysis are scarce. HBPM is an important tool in the regular monitoring of blood pressure (BP) and in patient's involvement in its long-term self-management. Nurses have an important role here and their involvement in the process is essential. Nurses must be aware of the latest recommendations as well as they should teach, train, guide and supervise patients. This chapter summarizes information about CKD and hypertension, the importance of measuring blood pressure at home in CKD and describes nursing interventions in this field. Nurses have a role in enabling patients to optimize their self-management skills. Nurse-delivered interventions have been shown to contribute to improved patient outcomes. Nurses can educate patients about proper blood pressure monitoring techniques at home, and also interpreting and evaluating the results and managing the therapeutic regimen. Evidence shows the effects of interventions performed by nurses in improving and controlling BP, such as teaching, training, counseling, motivational interview, coaching, nurse–patient relationship, communication, negotiation, and support.

Keywords: home blood pressure, self-management, nurse interventions, chronic kidney disease, health gains

1. Introduction

It is worldwide recognized the impact of kidney disease in economy and society. In developed countries, the costs associated with dialysis treatment and transplantation consume 2 to 3% of the health budget. On the other hand, in middle and low-income countries the accessibility to kidney function replacement treatments is low [1].

Chronic kidney disease (CKD) is considered a public health problem and has a significant weight in the context of chronic diseases. This disease affects around 850 million people worldwide, with one in ten adults having chronic kidney disease [2].

All stages of the disease - 1 to 5 -, are associated with increased risk of cardiovascular morbidity, premature mortality and quality of life decrease [3].

Considering the weight of hypertension, cardiovascular disease and diabetes mellitus in the increase of CKD, it is crucial to be concerned with its management.

2. Chronic kidney disease and hypertension

There is a complex association between CKD and hypertension due to a cause-effect relationship, in which both hypertension and CKD have a risk factor sharing relationship, being that one may be the cause or consequence of the other. Every year the number of people diagnosed with CKD due to hypertension increases by 10%.

The literature states that 5% of CKD are due to hypertension. It is highlighted that hypertension is more common in glomerular diseases, but the incidence of this clinical condition differs according to the histological characteristics of the disease. Membranoproliferative glomerulonephritis and segmental and focal glomerulosclerosis forms have a higher incidence of hypertension than membranous forms and IgA glomerulopathy. **Table 1** shows the prevalence of hypertension in different chronic renal diseases [4].

The evidence supports that the prevalence of hypertension increases as kidney function deteriorates in CRD, with a progressive decrease in the glomerular filtration rate [5].

Several studies have shown that hypertension is an independent risk factor for end-stage renal disease (ESRD), contributing to the disease itself and its progression [6, 7].

Cardiovascular disease is the leading cause of death in CKD, which in turn, increases the risk of long-term cardiovascular events [8].

When compared to the general population, the prevalence of hypertension is higher in people with CKD, constituting the factor with the greatest impact on the progression and outcome of kidney disease [9].

It is not yet known the exact mechanism that causes hypertension in CKD, nor has been isolated any factor responsible for its establishment. It is theorized that there are several mechanisms that, acting together, contribute to increased blood pressure, such as the progressive loss of sodium excretion with the consequent volume overload, the excessive activity of the renin-angiotensin system, the disproportionate increase in sympathetic activity, secondary hyperparathyroidism, the reduction of nitric oxide synthesis and the high endothelin levels, among others [10, 11].

Chronic kidney disease	% of hypertension patients
Glomerular diseases	
Segmental and focal glomerulosclerosis	75–80
Membranoproliferative glomerulonephritis	65–70
Diabetic nephropathy	65–70
Membranous nephropathy	40–50
Mesangial proliferative glomerulonephritis	35–40
IgA nephropathy	30
Minimal change disease	20–30
Polycystic kidney disease	60
Chronic interstitial nephritis	35

Table 1.
Hypertension prevalence in CKD patients.

Observational studies report an increased risk of development and rapid progression of CKD in cases of uncontrolled blood pressure [12].

Failure to treat hypertension is associated with harmful effects such as left ventricular hypertrophy, dilated cardiomyopathy and accelerated deterioration of renal function, among other causes [10].

According to Kidney Disease Improving Global Outcomes (KDIGO), international organizations (such as National Kidney Foundation Kidney Disease Outcomes Quality Initiative - NKF KDODQI; Eighth Joint National Committee published - JNC 8) committed to the prevention and treatment of hypertension recommend non-pharmacological measures along with pharmacological measures in the prevention and treatment of this disease [13, 14].

According to these organizations, health professionals are responsible for early detection of the disease and monitoring of risk factors.

The disease can progress slowly due to the gradual loss of the nephrons, and in its initial stages it goes unnoticed, only being identified when symptoms appear.

The purpose of screening and monitoring the disease in the early stages is to delay its progression to ESRD, a condition that leads to the need for renal replacement therapy.

Only a minority of patients with hypertension have blood pressure within the accepted target values (systolic blood pressure less than 140 mmHg, diastolic blood pressure less than 90 mmHg). The main causes for the lack of blood pressure control are related to low knowledge of the problem and lack of screening for hypertension in the population [15].

In the context of non-pharmacological measures, European Society of Cardiology makes clear the urgent need to promote preventive actions, mentioning that blood pressure measurement is a simple, non-invasive and low-cost technique, especially if considering the costs of treating hypertension and associated complications.

Regarding hypertension and kidney disease, there is no consensus among the authors about what the reference values should be. This is an issue that remains in debate despite recent recommendations and the publication of the clinical trials SPRINT, ACCORD, among others [16, 17].

The European Society of Hypertension and the European Society of Cardiology (ESH/ESC) recommend target blood pressure values below 140/90 mmHg for blood pressure measurements in a clinical setting. However, in the presence of proteinuria, these values drop to 130/80 mmHg as a reference. Similar recommendations are indicated by the JNC-8, suggesting target blood pressure values below 140/90 mmHg for the general population, disregarding the recommendations of SPRINT study, which suggests blood pressure values below 130/80 mmHg for patients at increased risk of cardiovascular events, including patients with CKD [18].

Target blood pressure values have changed over time. The literature shows that the target blood pressure value acceptable for patients with CKD is 130/80 mmHg [19]. The latest guidelines of the European Society of Hypertension and the European Society of Cardiology published in 2018 recommend a target SBP (Systolic Blood Pressure) value of 130–139 mmHg and DBP (Diastolic Blood Pressure) of 70–79 mmHg for patients with CKD. But there is not a unanimous view among scientific community on this issue [20, 21].

Vital for the success of the blood pressure prevention and control programs is the participation of the patient/family.

Health care, as integrating element of praxis, which takes place during the course of the chronic disease, calls for the participation of all stakeholders in the care process and for the investment in patients' education, enabling them to understand their health needs and become co-responsible for their health and well-being [22].

Everybody should to be part of an active citizenship stance based on education and training. Care must focus on the needs of the patient, it is important to know their level of mastery in response to the needs considered significant at any stage of the disease pathway [23].

3. Home blood pressure measurement

Blood pressure self-monitoring has been proposed as a strategy to improve hypertension control. Although the results of previous clinical trials on blood pressure measurement in the adjustment of hypertensive therapy and in the control of hypertension are inconsistent, the results of TASMINH4 demonstrated that 90% of eligible participants revealed that they wanted to take an active role in self-monitoring of blood pressure [24].

However, the importance of new studies in this area is highlighted, mainly studies involving risk groups, including patients with CKD in the advanced stage of the disease [25].

Hypertension is common in CKD patients, with a prevalence of around 60% to 90%, depending on the stage and cause of the disease, and is responsible for high cardiovascular morbidity and mortality. In this context, blood pressure control is a key measure [10].

HBPM is easier than ambulatory blood pressure measurement and, therefore, can be an important tool for blood pressure control in combination with other measures.

In this regard, Sanghavi, & Vassalotti emphasize that measuring blood pressure at home is a mean of reducing the burden of medication in individuals with "white coat hypertension", that is defined as the increase in blood pressure in the clinical context and maintenance of normal values at home. And, therefore, a means of improving the therapeutic compliance of hypertensive patients [26].

The authors also add that HBPM offers the patient a means to monitor the effectiveness of the medication and acts as a positive reinforcement, as shown by a study carried out in Spain. Of the 250 participants, 92% of the individuals in the experimental group (home blood pressure measurement) adhered to the antihypertensive regime, against 74% in the control group.

They concluded that HBPM is simple and not expensive. Besides, it offers more information to the practitioner, allowing more informed clinical decisions. It also promotes the involvement of the patient and the commitment of the health team, including nurses.

The evidence that shows the benefits of HBPM compared to measuring blood pressure in the clinical setting. Namely in improving blood pressure control, in reducing "white coat hypertension" events and in cardiovascular risk prediction [27–29].

The diagnosis of "white coat hypertension" is important because one of the consequences of this situation is overtreatment [30].

CKD patients with "white coat hypertension" have a lower cumulative risk of progressing to ESRD, so home blood pressure monitoring is essential. On the other side, renal patients have a high prevalence of masked hypertension, defined as normal blood pressure values in the clinical setting and high blood pressure values at home or ambulatory. This situation puts them at risk of organ damage, cardiovascular events and tends to evolve to ESRD [31].

HBPM allows a complementary assessment of daytime blood pressure variation, commonly seen in chronic kidney patients [32, 33].

Self-measurement of blood pressure at home is therefore an alternative for measuring blood pressure. Besides providing a more accurate assessment of blood pressure, it offers the possibility of having regular measurements in conditions closer to the patients' daily lives [34].

It is recognized by the scientific community that the measurement of blood pressure in the clinical context does not accurately reflect the blood pressure of each individual (due to changes in circadian rhythm and in the environment). It is thus necessary to create alternative methods whose main goal is to enable a closer assessment of the patient's values, because it takes place in a natural context, in the patient's natural environment [35].

Therefore, the self-monitoring of blood pressure at home becomes a tool to be incorporated into the self-care of CKD patients, through which the person has control over the process. This action makes the patient co-responsible for their health. This is a simple and important measure in preventing progression to ESRD, but it is nevertheless a complement to blood pressure measurement in the clinical context [36].

The negative individual, social, and economic consequences of not controlling blood pressure are evident. But these effects can be positive when enhanced by the self-management of hypertension.

The main negative effects resulting from the lack of blood pressure control in CKD patients call for the development of self-care interventions that result in behavior modification and optimization of hypertension control.

This issue is evident in the study by Humpherys et al., which, through a multifaceted intervention approach, optimized blood pressure values in proteinuric CKD patients and unproteinuric CKD patients. For that, the authors run 4 projects, which occurred in different practices, established chronologically in different periods of time. The percentage of patients with self-care behaviors for blood pressure management within the recommended target values increased from 34% to 74% in project 1, from 60% to 83% in project 2, from 68% to 71% in project 3 and 63% to 76% in project 4. Both groups (proteinuric and unproteinuric CKD patients) were able to reach the recommended target blood pressure values. The group of unproteinuric patients achieved blood pressure values below 140/90 mmHg and the group of proteinuric patients reached values of blood pressure below 130/80 mmHg. In this context, the authors concluded that this type of intervention proves to be an asset in reducing long-term complications resulting from suboptimization of blood pressure control [22].

The analysis of the systematic literature review carried out by Gallagher, et al. shows us the positive effects of educational interventions in reducing high blood pressure. The benefits of health education interventions in lowering blood pressure in chronic kidney patients were confirmed. As well as their potential in reducing cardiovascular events and delaying the progression of the disease [37].

Given that nurses have a pivotal role in promoting self-care behaviors in all aspects of care, including (1) problem identification, (2) diagnosis, (3) intervention, (4) evaluation and (5) follow-up, it is essential to highlight the interventions developed in the context of high blood pressure control in chronic kidney patients.

According to the literature, the possible causes of blood pressure control in this target group are associated with a reduction in self-care behaviors in relation to the consumption of salt, the practice of physical exercise and the adherence to medication. The overlook of these behaviors leads to hypertension. In this context, non-pharmacological interventions are relevant, along with pharmacological measures [38].

4. The role of nursing education in promoting patient's kidney self-care capacities

Health education, as a field for knowledge production, assumes a privileged relationship with active citizenship, providing patient/family with the possibility of making informed decisions and acting in collaboration with the health team.

Assuming the empowerment speech as a key element of the care action, which is shaped at the border between the biomedical model and the model of care centred on the patient, Orem's theory of self-care fits in this context. Especially when it is intended to establish partnerships and promote self-care behaviors in the prevention and control of hypertension in patients with CKD through an educational intervention.

According to Orem, the individual is an active subject, but in a situation of illness, his capacity for self-care can be reduced due to his inefficiency in relation to the condition that affects him [39].

In 2013, the World Health Organization (WHO) defined self-care as the ability of individuals, families and the community to promote health, prevent disease and stay healthy. The partnership with healthcare professionals to deal with the disease and disabilities arises when individuals are unable to meet some or all of the needs for self-care, due to a lack of knowledge, disability or perception of their diminished health status.

Nurses act as a resource for the patient, developing helping methods in order to overcome or compensate health-related limitations, leading the patient to undertake actions to regulate their own functioning and development. The intervention is carried out according to a diagnostic and intervention process. It starts with needs assessment, identification of motivation to learn and, in partnership with the patient and/or family, establishment of the goals to be achieved. In this process the nurse can direct, guide, provide support and teach [39].

CKD patients need to undertake a range of complex activities, such as monitoring blood pressure, blood glucose, introducing changes in diet, adhering to therapy, avoiding nephrotoxic substances and practicing physical exercise [40].

It is internationally recognized that disease self-management is now an essential aspect of the health system. The implementation of a disease self-management plan based on negotiated complementary actions, allows the process participants to rediscover the conditions (knowledge and skills) to satisfy their needs. With the aging of population, families assume an increasing importance in the daily management of the disease. Therefore, families and patients are the clients of health professionals and the expression of their interests must be taken into account [41].

There are many difficulties for active participation of individuals in the management of their disease due to lack of knowledge and skills to deal with the disease. Therefore, between unawareness and fears, people's behavior can take two directions: control or ignore the problem. In either cases, nurses have a predominant support role in making people aware of their potential, leading them to develop and put that potential at the service of the disease.

Health education is a strategy to be followed, as it constitutes a teaching, instruction and training tool in order to guide the patient and their families to face a new situation in the management and prevention of the disease.

It is true that CKD patients have the same characteristics as the general population in terms of self-care behaviors in controlling blood pressure, following a healthy diet and regular physical exercise. However, it is no less true that CKD disease, due to its complexity and need for intervention in all of the stages, requires specific intervention and monitoring actions along the path of the disease.

As CKD is an asymptomatic disease, especially in the early stages, it means that patients with CKD, because they are unaware of their situation, do not seek information. It is also a fact that the low perception of susceptibility is associated with low levels of literacy and, consequently, with a reduced perception of the risk of developing the disease [40].

This discouraging picture highlights important gaps regarding the patient's monitoring plan. In this context, innovative and complementary practices are needed to implement an individualized monitoring program based on the patient's real problems, both in hospitals and in primary health care. As a reference, we identify health education projects developed in specialized hospital consultations, or even in the wards, based on information, instruction and training techniques aimed at this population.

The question that arises is: what directions can be pursued to achieve these goals?

Firstly, it is essential to identify and accurately assess self-care behaviors, regarding blood pressure monitoring at home and levels of activation in disease management in its various stages. Secondly, the implementation of an intervention that promotes knowledge, skills and patient activation in the disease management. That is, providing the means to enable patients to make informed decisions, make a self-monitoring and self-assessment of their condition and implement strategies to solve some problems that arise [42].

Indeed, in the context of CKD research, self-management interventions are on the top of the agenda when it comes to preventing disease progression [43]. For example, Havas et al. indicates that chronic kidney patients reported the need to learn how self-manage their disease and to integrate self-management behaviors into their daily lives [44].

In this context, the education process is a fundamental tool. For it to be successful it is important to take into account the motivation, the literacy level, the patient activation in disease management and the patient/health professional relationship [45].

Activation is an interactive process and consists of the patient's ability to actively participate in disease management, to assume an active behavior in favor of a passive attitude. Several factors take action in this process, such as the patient's motivation, beliefs, knowledge and abilities/skills to perform [46].

Activated patients have higher scores for participation in disease self-management, namely blood pressure monitoring, healthy eating habits, physical exercise, smoking cessation, etc., when compared to those who are not [47].

Activation exists in a continuum in which the patient moves between four levels, depending on state of health, self-confidence, motivation to get involved and circumstances of life.

The four levels are:

1. **Beliefs:** activated patients **believe** they have a fundamental role in disease self-management and health status maintenance, collaborating with health professionals.

2. **Trust and knowledge to take action:** activated patients have **knowledge and confidence** in disease self-management.

3. **Take action:** activated patients **have the skills** to manage their health condition.

4. **Maintaining action:** activated patients **maintain** their functionality even if exposed to high levels of stress [48].

Along with the concept of patient activation, the concept of perceived efficacy gains relevance in the disease self-management. To the previous ones, demographic characteristics (age, gender, education) and clinical characteristics (cognitive and physical capacity) are added.

Perceived self-efficacy refers to the person's perception of their own ability to perform a certain activity in order to achieve a goal or result. According to Bandura, it is important for people to believe that they are able to successfully develop a certain action, because that will be the guarantee of getting involved and adopting goals for that purpose [49].

Bandura also defines how much effort a person will need and how long it will last when faced with difficulties and negative experiences. There is a tendency to avoid situations that may exceed the limit of the person's capabilities and to deal with those that the person thinks are solvable. The person tends to distance from situations with high levels of demand, offering the most varied justifications [50].

In this way, different scores for perception of self-efficacy can increase or decrease the motivation for action, with higher self-efficacy scores corresponding to better health. Previous research has shown this relationship, in addition to showing that high self-efficacy was associated with positive changes in health behaviors [49].

Several studies in nephrology field have found an association between high levels of perceived self-efficacy and health gains in groups of hemodialysis patients, regarding weight control improvement between dialysis sessions, reducing hospitalizations, amputations and improving quality of life [51].

Taking into account the international scenario, hypertension represents a burden for global disease context. Thus, standardized blood pressure measurement is essential for diagnosis and blood pressure management [36].

Lopez-vargas et al. showed that patients with CKD in the most advanced stages have low levels of knowledge about the associated risk factors, including hypertension and its management. The authors found that 54% of the patients received information on blood pressure monitoring, adherence to therapy and food preparation. They also identified that nurses had the main role of educators in 73% of the necessary studies. The results indicated that of the 54% of the patients involved in disease self-management, 31% had their blood pressure controlled [52].

The interventions that most contributed to the effectiveness of the process were: teaching practical skills, workshops, follow-up patient on a regular basis and negotiating goals to achieve.

Patients involved in blood pressure monitoring at home learn to understand the connection between measuring and controlling blood pressure and more easily adhere to strategies that contribute to controlling blood pressure, specifically diet, exercise and adherence to therapy. This attitude towards the disease shows improvements in health status [53].

For Wanchai & Armer nurses can help the patient to improve their self-care skills [54]. The question is: how to do it?

Returning to Orem's theory, the authors mention that there are three classifications of nursing systems to meet the self-care requisites of the patient: wholly compensatory system, partially compensatory system and the supportive-educative system. Regarding the first system, nurses need to completely replace the individual due to the inability to self-care. In the second system, a patient can meet some self-care requisites but needs a nurse to help meet other needs. In the supportive-educative system, a patient can meet self-care requisites but needs assistance with decision making, behavior control, or knowledge acquisition skills, so nurses teach, train and support the patient for self-care. Often the patient is unable to perform his activities because he does not have the necessary knowledge to perform them. According to Orem, in some situations, the patient needs the nurse's guidance to carry out the self-care action and in other situations he needs to learn the techniques to be able to perform them.

The authors mention other methods of training the patient for self-care, promoted by nurses, such as coaching, stimulating the patient's participation and establishing of therapeutic relationship.

The authors add the motivational interview as a strategy to motivate the patient to change specific behaviors. They also report that review studies have shown the effectiveness of this method in changing behaviors for healthy lifestyles. Other authors have stated that this type of approach is useful in situations where the patient is less motivated to assume self-care or in situations where the patient not yet prepared to take charge of his illness condition.

In the context of health education, giving educational materials can help the patient in the learning process. However, it is necessary to pay attention to the patient's abilities in terms of reading and comprehension to avoid bad decisions about self-care. The demonstration and training blood pressure measurement in different methods involving the technique of blood pressure measurement at home should be promoted. Additional resources such as videos, access to websites dedicated to this subject or leaflets demonstrating the technique, may be useful in demonstrating blood pressure monitoring at home.

Nurses play an important role in this process, helping the patients to select and understand the best method for themselves [55].

Nurses should inform the patient about the recommended schedule for blood pressure monitoring at home. According to the European Hypertension Society Working Group, blood pressure should be taken twice in the morning and twice in the afternoon [56].

In some experts' opinion, blood pressure self-monitoring over a long period may allow a more accurate assessment of blood pressure stability and increase the patient's commitment to treatment.

Nurses should discuss with patients the importance of blood pressure self-management. Therefore, an important element in this whole process is the communication established between the health professional and the patient. Feedback should be maintained even when the professional is not on duty. The patient should be able to communicate with the healthcare professional via telephone, fax and e-mail. There are also other ways of data communication, namely through stored data in devices, mobile phone applications (smartphone applications) and internet.

Nurses can help the patient to obtain health gains through adequate training in blood pressure measuring methodology and interpreting the values obtained in blood pressure monitoring at home.

To this purpose, nurses should explain and demonstrate the technique to the patient and inform about the recommended devices [57]. The **Table 2** shows the Society of Cardiology and the European Society of Hypertension recommendations regarding blood pressure measurement at home.

Regarding device selection, literature indicates that the recommended devices for HBPM are the automatic oscillometric arm devices. This kind of equipment is more user-friendly and requires less skills when compared to manual devices.

Electronic arm devices for BP measurement, especially those that allow the storage, transmission or printing measuring data, should be preferred for HBPM. It is also crucial that patients make sure that the devices they acquire have been validated according to recommended criteria. The European Society for Hypertension Working Group on Blood Pressure Monitoring has developed a protocol applicable to most BP measuring devices available on the market. The European Society of Hypertension supported the creation of a website where updated lists of validated BP measurement devices are published (www.dableeducational). The British

Environment	**Comfortable environment temperature** **Quiet and noiseless environment**
Patient	Training in blood pressure measurement technique is required **Measurement conditions and procedures:** • Patients should be relaxed, in a seating position with their backs supported and uncrossed legs; • Wait for 5 minutes at rest before beginning BP measurements. Patients should remain alone where the blood pressure is measured; • The bladder must be empty; • Do not eat or smoke within 30 minutes of BP measuring; • Do not exercise in the 60 minutes before BP measurement; • Do not speak before and during the BP measurement. **Arm Position and support** • The arm should be resting on a table with the palm facing up, positioned at the level of the heart. The arm on which the blood pressure will be assessed should be free of clothing, preferably bare. **Arm selection** • Blood pressure should be, preferably, measured on the right arm; • The left arm should be used if BP values are higher than in the right arm or due to an abnormality or some circumstance that indicates against its use. In the case CKD patients, it is essential to check for arteriovenous fistulas (AVFs) or arteriovenous grafts (AVGs). Do not assess the blood pressure in the access arm; • Record blood pressure assessment arm is also required.
Blood pressure measurement devices	**Blood pressure cuff size** • Before using the BP measuring device ensure that the cuff dimensions are adequate; • In relation to the length, the bladder inside the cuff should encircle 80 to 100% of the arm; the bladder width should be 40 to 50% of arm circumference. **Blood pressure cuff position** • It should be 2–3 cm above the cubital fossa, at the level of the heart; • At each BP measurement the cuff should be wrapped around the arm with the central area placed over the brachial artery. **Time and frequency for BP measurement** • Three consecutive readings in the morning (in fasting and before taking the medication) in the afternoon and evening; • Repeat the measurement with 1–2 minutes interval between; • Record the values obtained.

Table 2.
Recommendations for HBPM.

Hypertension Society (www.bhsoc.org) also publishes information on device validation.

In Herber, et al., it is essential that the patient and family have coping strategies to deal with the disease and complications. The authors highlight the role of regular home visits in establishing a therapeutic relationship. In these visits, nurses can support and teach the patient and family to manage the therapeutic regimen, increase levels of knowledge about the disease and self-care behaviors, as well as guide the resources available in the community [58].

For Coates et al., the management of the disease is challenging, both for the patient and his relatives, as well as for health professionals, as it requires a change in the philosophy of care. The paradigm change demands the active involvement of the patient in decisions and problem solving. In this context, new strategies are required to make the patient responsible for the management of his health [59].

Negotiation is, thus, an important strategy to prevent the patient from adopting a passive attitude and, at the same time, to equip the patient with the necessary skills and abilities for disease management [60].

Advice and support in changing daily routines are essential for the control of HTA [61].

Blood pressure self-monitoring makes patients more aware of their pressure values and leads them to commit themselves more actively in their therapeutic plan.

In summary, self-care is an essential component for chronic disease management and, in the case of CKD, is certainly a sine qua non condition. The evolutionary path of CKD brings with it a growing number of daily self-care activities for the individual, such as deciding what to do, undertaking self-care activities related to disease monitoring and putting a strong increase in the investment of healthy behaviors, including blood pressure control, diet and exercise, among others.

The health gains for the patient consist of increased quality of life, empowerment, success in lifestyle changes due to active role and involvement in disease management. The change in perception of hypertension can encourage the patient to comply with therapy and make the necessary lifestyle changes [62].

5. Conclusion

The main objective of HBPM is to prevent and delay morbidity, mortality and organ damage. To achieve this goal, it is essential to implement pharmacological and non-pharmacological measures, including: regular blood pressure measuring throughout life at home. This self-care behavior results in gains for the patient as it has been shown in CKD patients. Adequate blood pressure control reduces the rate of decline in kidney function and cardiovascular morbidity and. In this context, HBPM is important for the effective management of hypertension in this group with compromised kidney function [27, 63].

Nurses play an important role in patient empowerment by accompanying, teaching, training and informing about hypertension and the additional measures needed to achieve the expected result: blood pressure control and quality of life. The establishment and maintenance of a model of care based on cooperation between health professionals and the patient is the key to success.

Conflict of interest

The authors declare no conflict of interest.

Author details

Dilar Costa* and Filipa Aguiar
North Lisbon Hospital Center, Lisbon, Portugal

*Address all correspondence to: dilarcosta@gmail.com

References

[1] Macário, F. Some reflections on renal care. Port J Nephrol Hypert. 2019; 33 (4): 209-211. DOI: 10.32932/pjnh.2020.01.043.

[2] Carney, E.F. The impact of chronic kidney disease on global health. Nat Rev Nephrol. 2020; 16: 251. DOI: 10.1038/s41581-020-0268-7.

[3] Hill NR, Fatoba ST, Oke JL, Hirst JA, O'Callaghan CA, Lasserson DS, et al. Global Prevalence of Chronic Kidney Disease – A Systematic Review and Meta-Analysis. PLoS One [Internet]. 2016 [cited 2020 Nov 27]; 11 (7):1-18. Available from: https://www.ncbi.nlm.nih.gov/pmc/articles/PMC4934905/ DOI: 10.1371/journal.pone.0158765.

[4] Woronik V. Hipertensão e doenças primárias renais. Hiperativo. 1998; 5 (4): 253-60. http://departamentos.cardiol.br/dha/revista/5-4/hipertensao.pdf.

[5] Tedla F, Brar A, Browne R, Brown C. Hypertension in chronic kidney disease: navigating the evidence. Int J Hypertens. 2011; 2011 (1324805): 1-9. DOI:10.4061/2011/132405.

[6] Morgado E, Neves PL. Hypertension and chronic kidney disease: Cause and consequence – therapeutic considerations. In Babaei Editor. In Antihypertensive drugs [Internet]. Iran: Tabriz University of Medical Sciences; 2012 [cited 2020 Oct 26] Available from: https://www.intechopen.com/books/antihypertensive-drugs/hypertension-in-chronic-kidney-disease-cause-and-consequence-therapeutic-considerations-

[7] Ravara M, Deferrari MRL, Vettoretti S, Deferrari G. Importance of blood pressure control in chronic kidney disease. J AM Soc Nephrol. 2006; 17 (4 Suppl 2): S98-103. DOI: 10.1681/ASN.2005121319.

[8] Bikbov B, Purcell CA, Levey AS, Smith M, Abdoli A, Abebe M, et al. Global, regional, and national burden of chronic kidney disease, 1990-2017: a systematic analysis for the Global Burden of Disease Study 2017. Lancet. 2020; 395 (10225): 709-733. DOI: 10.1016/s0140-6736(20)30045-3.

[9] Kim IY, Song SH. Blood pressure measurement in patients with chronic kidney disease: from clinical trial to clinical practice. Kidney Res Clin Pract. 2019; 38 (2): 138-140. DOI: 10.23876/J.Krcp.19.032.

[10] Ku E, Lee BJ, Wei J, Weir MR. Hypertension in CKD: Core Curriculum 2019. Am J Kidney Dis. 2019; 74 (1): 120-131. DOI: 10.1053/j.ajkd.2018.12.044.

[11] Zanatta CM, Canani LH, Silveiro SP, Burttiet L, Nabinger G, Gross JL. Arq Bras Endocrinol Metab. 2008; 52 (4): 581-8. DOI: 10.1590/S0004-27302008000400003.

[12] Webster AC, Nagler EV, Morton RL, Masson P. Chronic Kidney disease. Lancet. 2017; 389 (16): 1238-52. DOI: 10.1016/S0140-6736(16)32064-5.

[13] Kidney Disease Improving Global Outcomes (KDIGO) CKD Work Group. KDIGO Clinical Practice Guideline for the Management of Blood Pressure in Chronic Kidney Disease. 2012; 2 (5): 337-414.

[14] Eight Join National Committee (JNC8) JNC8 Guidelines for the Management of Hypertension in Adults. Am Fam Physician. 2014; 90 (7): 503-4.

[15] Beaney T, Burrell LM, Castillo RR, Charchar FJ, Cro S, Damasceno A, et al. Measurement month 2018: a pragmatic global screening campaign to raise awareness of blood pressure by the International Society of Hypertension.

Eur Heart J. 2019; 40 (25): 2006-2017. DOI: 10.1093/eurheartj/ehz300.

[16] SPRINT Research Group. A randomized trial of intensive versus standard blood-pressure control. SPRINT study. N Engl Med. 2015; 373 (22): 2103-2116. DOI: 10.1056/NEJMoa1511939. Epub 2015 Nov 9.

[17] ACCORD Study Group. Effects of Intensive blood-pressure control in type 2 diabetes mellitus. N Engl Med. 2010; 362 (17): 1575-85. DOI: 10.1056/NEJMoa1001286. Epub 2010 Mar 14.

[18] Wyatt CM, Chertow GM. Clinical trials of intensive versus less intensive control of hypertension: HOPE or HYPE? Kidney Int. 2016; 90 (3): 460-2. DOI: 10.1016/j.kint.2016.06.021.

[19] Chang AR, Lóser M, Mahotra R, Appel LJ. Blood pressure goals in patients with CKD. A review of evidence and guidelines. Clin J Am soc Nephrol. 2019; 14 (1): 161-69. DOI: 10.2215/CJN.07440618.

[20] O'Brien E, Pickering T, Asmar R, Myers M, Parati G, Staessen J, et al. Working Group on Blood Pressure Monitoring of the European Society of Hypertension International Protocol for validation of blood pressure measuring devices in adults. Blood Press Monit. 2002; 1 (3): 3-17. DOI: 10.1097/00126097-200202000-00002.

[21] Williams B, Mancia G, Spiering W, Rosei, EA, Azizi M, Burnier M, et al. 2018 ESC/ESH Guidelines for the management of arteria hypertension: The Task Force for the management of arterial hypertension of the European Society of Cardiology (ESC) and the European Society of Hypertension (ESH). Guidelines for the management of arterial hypertension. European Heart Journal. 2018; 39 (33): 3021-3104. DOI: 10.1093/eurheartj/ehy339.

[22] Humphreys J, Harvey G, Hegarty J. Improving CKD diagnosis and blood pressure control in primary care: a tailored multifaceted quality improvement programme. Nephron Extra. 2017; 7 (1): 18-32. DOI: 10.1159/000458712.

[23] Nunes JW, Greene JH, Wallston K, Eden S, Shintani A, Elasy T, et al. Pilot study of a physician-delivered education tool to increase patient knowledge about CKD. Am J Kidney Dis. 2013; 62 (1), 23-32. DOI: 10.1053/j.ajkd.2013.01.023.

[24] McManus RJ, Mant J, Haque MS, Bray EP, Bryan S, Greenfield SM, et al. Effect of self-monitoring and self-titration on systolic blood pressure in hypertensive patients at high risk of cardiovascular disease: the TASMIN – SR randomized clinical trial. JAMA. 2014; 312 (8); 799-808. DOI: 10.1001/jama.2014.10057.

[25] Tyson, CC, Wyatt CM. There's no place like home: is self-monitoring beneficial in hypertension management? Kidney Int. 2018: 94 (3): 450-2. DOI: 10.1016/j.kint.2018.06.021.

[26] Sanghavi S, Vassalotti JÁ. Pratical use of blood pressure monitoring in chronic kidney disease. Cardiorenal Med. 2014; 4 (2): 113-122. DOI: 10.1159/000363114.

[27] Ward AM, Takahashi O, Stevens R, Heneghan C. Home measurement of blood pressure and cardiovascular disease: systematic review and meta-analysis of prospective studies. J Hypertens. 2012; 30 (3), 449-456. DOI: 10.1097/HJH.0b013e32834e4aed.

[28] Agarwal R. Ambulatory blood pressure and cardiovascular events in chronic kidney disease. Semin Nephrol. 2007; 27 (5), 538-43. DOI: 10.1016/j.semnephrol.2007.07.001.

[29] Bobrie G, Chatellier G, Genes N, Clerson P, Vaur L, Vaisse B, et al. Cardiovascular prognosis of "masked hypertension" detected by blood

pressure self-measurement in elderly treated hypertensive patients. JAMA. 2004; 291 (11): 1342-9. DOI: 10.1001/jama.291.11.1342.

[30] Huang Y, Huang W, Mai W, Xiaoyan C, An D, Liu Z, et al. White-coat hypertension is a risk factor for cardiovascular disease and total mortality. J Hypertens. 2017; 35 (4): 677-688. DOI: 10.1097/HJH.0000000000001226.

[31] Agarwal R, Anderson MJ, Bishu K, Saha C. Home blood pressure monitoring improves the diagnosis of hypertension in hemodialysis patients. Kidney Int. 2006; 69 (5): 900-6. DOI: 10.1038/sj.ki.5000145.

[32] Cunha C, Pereira S, Fernandes JC, Dias VP. 24-hour ambulatory blood pressure monitoring in chronic kidney disease and its influence on treatment. Port J Nephrol Hypertens. [Internet]. 2017 [cited 2020 Oct 15]; 31 (1): 31-6. Available from: http://www.scielo.mec.pt/pdf/nep/v31n1/31n1a03.pdf.

[33] Drawz PE, Abdalla M, Rahman M. Blood pressure measurement: clinic, home, ambulatory, and beyond. Am J kidney Dis. 2012; 60 (3): 449-62. DOI: 10.1053/j.ajkd.2012.01.026.

[34] Pinto, CAM. A gestão da pessoa com hipertensão arterial na Unidade Móvel de Saúde. [master's thesis on the internet]. Viseu (Portugal): Instituto Politécnico de Viseu; 2016 [cited 2020 Oc 9]. 182 p. Available from: https://repositorio.ipv.pt/bitstream/10400.19/3338/1/C%c3%a1tiaAlexandraMarquesPinto%20DM.pdf.

[35] Mancia G, Backer GD, Dominiczak A, Cifkova R, Fagard R, Germano G, et al. 2007 Guidelines for the management of arterial hypertension: the task force for the management of arterial hypertension of the European Society of Cardiology (ESC). J Hypertens. 2007; 25 (6): 1105-87. DOI: 10.1097/HJH.0b013e3281fc975a.

[36] Hamrahian, SM, Falkner B. Hypertension in Chronic Kidney Disease. Adv Exp Med Biol. [Internet]. 2016 [cited 2020 Nov 10]; 307-325. Available from: 10.1007/5584_2016_84.

[37] Gallagher H, Lusignan S, Harris K, Cates C. Quality-improvement strategies for the management of hypertension in chronic kidney disease in primary care: a systematic review. Br J Gen Pract. 2010; 60 (575): e258-e265. DOI: 10.3399/bjgp10X502164.

[38] Agarwal R. Systolic hypertension in hemodialysis patients. Semin Dial. 2003; 16 (3): 208-13. DOI: 10.1046/j.1525-139x.2003.16041.x.

[39] Tomey AM, Alligood MR. Teóricas de Enfermagem e a sua obra. 5th ed. Loures, Portugal: Lusociência – Edições Técnicas e Científicas, Lda., 2004.

[40] Narva AS, Norton JM, Boulware LE. Educating patients about CKD: the path to self-management and patient-centered care. Clin J Am Soc Nephrolo. 2016; 11 (4): 694-703. DOI: 10.2215/CJN.07680715. Epub 2015 Nov 4.

[41] Grey M, Schulman-Green D, Knafl K, Reynolds NR. A revised self-and family management framework. Nurs Outlook. 2015; 63 (2): 162-70. DOI: 10.1016/j.outlook.2014.10.003. Epub 2014 Oct 15.

[42] Agena F, Silva, GCA, Pierin AMG. Monitorização residencial da pressão arterial: atualidades e papel do enfermeiro. Esc. Enferm. USP. [Internet] 2011 [cited 2020 Oct 18]; 45 (1): 252-7. Available from: https://doi.org/10.1590/S0080-62342011000100036.

[43] Tong A, Chando S, Crowe S, Manns B, Winkelmayer WC, Hemmelgarn B, et al. Research priority

setting in kidney disease: a systematic review. Am J Kidney Dis. 2015; 65 (5): 674-83. DOI: 10.1053/j.ajkd.2014.11.011.

[44] Havas K, Bonner A, Douglas C. Self-management support for people with chronic kidney disease: patient perspectives. J Renal Care. 2016: 42 (1): 7-14. DOI: 10.1111/jorc.12140. Epub 2015 Sep 24.

[45] Dias VLR. Tradução e Validação para Portugal do Patient Activation Measure 13 em pessoas com Diabetes Mellitus tipo 2. [master's thesis on the internet]. Lisboa (Portugal): Universidade Nova de Lisboa, Escola Nacional de Saúde Pública; 2014 [cited 2020 Nov 9]. 166 p. Available from: https://run.unl.pt/handle/10362/14757.

[46] Johnson ML, Zimmerman L, Welch JL, Hertzog M, Pozehl B, Plumb T. Patient Activation with knowledge, self-management, and confidence in Chronic Kidney Disease. J ren Care. 2016; 42 (1): 15-22. DOI: 10.1111/jorc.12142. Epub 2015 Nov 5.

[47] Rask KJ, Ziemer DC, Kohler SA, Hawley JN, Arinde FJ, Barnes CS. Patient activation is associated with healthy behaviors and ease in managing diabetes in an indigent population. Diabetes educ. 2009; 35 (4): 622-30. DOI: 10.1177/0145721709335004. Epub 2009 Apr 28.

[48] Hibbard JH, Stockard J, Mahoney ER, Tusler M. Development pf the patient activation measure (PAM): conceptualizing and measuring activation in patients and consumers. Health Serv Res. 2004; 39 (4 Pt 1): 1005-1026. DOI: 10.1111/j.1475-6773.2004.00269.x.

[49] Sbicigo JB, Teixeira MAP, Dias ACG, Dell'Aglio DD. Psychometric properties of the General Perceived Self-Efficacy Scale (EAGP). Psico [Internet] 2012 [cited 2020 Sept 12]; 43 (2): 139-146. Available from: https://revistaseletronicas.pucrs.br/ojs/index.php/revistapsico/article/view/11691

[50] Souza I, Souza MA de. Validação da Escala de Autoeficácia Geral Percebida. Ver Univ Rural Sér. Ciências Humanas. [Internet] 2004 [cited 2020 Oct 18]; 26 (1-2): 12-17. Available from: https://www.researchgate.net/publication/260338439_Validacao_da_Escala_de_Autoeficacia_Geral_Percebida.

[51] Wild MG, Wallston KA, Green JA, Beach LB, Umeukeje E, Nunes JAW, et al. The perceived medical condition self-management scale can be applied to patients with chronic kidney disease. Kidney Int. 2017; 92 (4): 972-8. DOI: 10.1016/j.kint.2017.03.018. Epub 2017 May 18.

[52] Lopez-Vargas PA, Tong A, Howell M, Craig JC. Educational interventions for patients with CKD: A Systematic Review. Am J Kidney Dis. 2016; 68 (3): 353-70. DOI: 10.1053/j.ajkd.2016.01.022.

[53] Obara T, Asayama TO, Metoki H, Inoue R, Kikuya M, Kato T, et al. Home blood pressure measurements associated with better blood pressure control; the J-HOME study. J Hum Hypertens. 2008; 22 (3): 197-204. DOI: 10.1038/sj.jhh.1002320. Epub 2008 Jan 3.

[54] Wanchai A, Armer JM. Promoting self-care capabilities of patients: nurses' roles. Nurs Health Care. [Internet] 2018 [cited 2020 Oct 24]; 7 (4): 1-3. Available from: https://juniperpublishers.com/jojnhc/pdf/JOJNHC.MS.ID.555719.pdf.

[55] Wilson FL, Mood DW, Risk J, Kershaw T. Evaluation of education materials using Orem's Self-Care Deficit Theory. Nurs Sci Q. 2003; 16 (1): 68-76. DOI: 10.1177/0894318402239069.

[56] O'Brien E, Coats A, Owens P, Petrie J, Padfield PL, Littler WA,

de Swiet M, Mee F. Use and interpretation of ambulatory blood pressure monitoring: recommendations of the British Hypertension Society. BMJ. 2000; 320 (7242):1128-34. DOI: 10.1136/bmj.320.7242.1128.

[57] Himmelfarb CRD, Commodore-Mensah Y. Expanding the role of nurses to improve hypertension care and control globally. Ann Glob Health. 2016; 82 (2): 243-53. DOI: 10.1016/j.aogh.2016.02.003.

[58] Herber OR, Schnepp W, Rieger MA. Developing a nurse-led education program to enhance self-care agency in leg ulcer patients. Nurs Sci Q. 2008; 21 (2): 150-5. DOI: 10.1177/0894318408314694.

[59] Coates VE. Role of nurses in supporting patients to self-management chronic conditions. Nurs Stand. 2017; 31 (38): 42-6. DOI: 10.7748/ns.2017.e10742.

[60] Coates VE, McCan A, Posner N, Gunn K, Seers K. 'Well, who do I phone? Preparing to urgent care: a challenge for patients and service providers alike. J Clin Nurs. 2015; 24 (15-16): 2152-63. DOI: 10.1111/jocn.12814. Epub 2015 Apr 16.

[61] Bos-Touwen I, Dijkkamp E, Kars M, trappenburg J, Wit N D, Schuurmans M. Potential for self-management in chronic care. Nurs Res. 2015; 64 (4): 282-90. DOI: 10.1097/NNR.0000000000000103.

[62] Ogedegbe O, Schoenthaler A. A systematic review of the effects of home blood pressure monitoring on medication adherence. J Clin Hypertens. 2006; 8 (3):174-80. DOI: 10.1111/j.1524-6175.2006.04872.x.

[63] Cappuccio FP, Kerry SM, Forbes L, Donald A. Blood pressure control by home monitoring: meta-analysis of randomised trials. BMJ. 2004: 329 (7458): 1-6. DOI: 10.1136/bmj.38121.684410.

Chapter 4

Features of Diagnostics and Differential Diagnostics of Chronic Heart Failure in Outpatient Clinics

Oleg Anatolievich Shtegman and Marina Mihailovna Petrova

Abstract

The Chapter contains information about the prevalence of heart failure (HF) among patients in outpatient practice. The causal structure of HF, the prevalence of risk factors for HF, and the occurrence of a reduced ejection fraction are described. It describes the frequency of overdiagnosis of HF, the disease most often simulating its symptoms. The difficulties associated with laboratory and instrumental diagnostics of this syndrome are discussed. A pharmacological test for differential diagnosis of the causes of dyspnea in patients with suspected HF is described. Information is provided on the incidence of depressive and anxiety among the patients with this disease.

Keywords: heart failure, prevalence, outpatient, diagnostics, differential diagnostics, pharmacological test, torasemide, depressive, anxiety

1. Introduction

Chronic HF is a common complication of cardiovascular diseases. The widespread prevalence of this pathology in the world in recent years has taken on the scale of an epidemic. Tens of millions of people around the world suffer from this disease. It can be made with the growing burden of obesity-related diseases and with the aging of the population [1]. Probably, it is also important to increase the survival rate after acute forms of coronary artery disease and increase the life expectancy of patients with HF. Diagnosis of chronic HF is a major clinical problem, especially in patients with comorbidities [2]. This Chapter aims to highlight the features of the diagnosis of HF in an outpatient setting.

2. The prevalence of heart failure among patients in outpatient practice

The reasons for visiting a polyclinic by patients are often acute diseases, the need for a health examination, or dispensary monitoring for chronic diseases. The cohort of such visitors does not accurately reflect the state of the population, but these are the people that outpatient doctors have to deal with.

Many variants of criteria for the diagnosis of heart failure in epidemiological studies have been developed. Their diversity highlights the inferiority of diagnostic methods. There are Framingham, Gothenburg, Boston, European society of cardiology criteria and others. We used a questionnaire proposed by the Russian society of heart failure specialists [3]. The questionnaire includes a question about the presence of shortness of breath, confirmation of myocardial damage by instrumental methods, taking diuretics, a known diagnosis of heart failure, and a decrease in the left ventricular ejection fraction of less than 50%. A positive answer to the first question and any subsequent question makes it likely that the patient has HF.

In a survey of 3,000 adults who consecutively applied to the outpatient clinic, it was found that 543 patients were suspected of heart failure. The recruitment of people in the study was carried out by age and gender groups identical to the population living in the city. Among people who visit an outpatient department, the clinical suspicion of heart failure among men is 12.3%, among women it reaches 22.9% [4]. At the same time, it is possible to confirm the presence of heart failure in 11.7% of outpatient patients. In 36.2% of outpatient visitors with suspected HF, the disease is not confirmed during further examination. These cases were 57% more common among women compared to men.

The specificity of the questionnaire used was 63.8%. Thus, after clinical screening for possible HF, additional methods should be used that exclude the situation of overdiagnosis.

The vast majority of patients (87%) have HF with preserved ejection fraction (EF). However, among hospitalized patients with heart failure, the ratio between preserved and reduced ejection fraction is approximately one to one [5].

3. The prevalence of risk factors of heart failure among patients in outpatient practice

An analysis of a sample of 3,000 outpatient visitors found that the prevalence of obesity among adult outpatient patients is 20% (95% CI: 18.6–21.4%). Obesity increased the likelihood of shortness of breath in men and women almost equally (the relative risk was 2.39 and 2.49, respectively). The prevalence of diabetes mellitus, according to the survey, among adult outpatient visitors is 5.9%. The prevalence of smoking and alcohol abuse among adult outpatient visitors is 35% and 12.4%, respectively. The prevalence of MI among adult outpatient patients is 4.7%. According to the survey, the prevalence of hypertension among adult outpatient visitors was 37.9%.

Hence, among the risk factors, arterial hypertension has the greatest population contribution to the development of HF. It was found that not only the presence and severity of arterial hypertension affected the development of HF, but also the duration of increased blood pressure. Thus, in patients with confirmed HF, dyspnea developed on average only 8.4 years after the onset of hypertension, and in patients with excluded HF, dyspnea occurred only 2.8 years later. That is, when assessing the probability of a connection between the appearance of shortness of breath, the exposure to hypertension should be taken into account.

4. The clinical diagnosis of heart failure

The diagnosis of chronic HF begins, of course, with the patient's complaints. Thanks to the existing complaints of the patient that he comes into our field of vision. However, the complaints are not specific. If the patient has a complex of manifestations of heart failure such as oedema, orthopnea, complaints of dyspnea, heaviness in the right hypochondrium, fatigue, then we will not be difficult to diagnose HF. But if we consider each of the signs of heart failure separately, it turns out that their specificity is quite low. And just such a situation is observed in the initial manifestations of heart failure. These patients, who have 1–2 manifestations, are the cornerstone of the diagnosis of initial forms of heart failure.

The most common manifestation of chronic heart failure is a complaint of shortness of breath. The sensitivity of this sign is close to 100%, but the specificity is only 17% [6]. When dyspnea is difficult for the patient to inhale, it has mostly inspiratory character. The shortness of breath is quite stereotypical. It cannot be there for a while, then disappear and reappear spontaneously. Without a treatment it constantly progresses as a rule. In patients with limited mobility, dyspnea may not appear during exercise, but may debut at night in a horizontal position. Short-acting nitrates and diuretics can have a good effect on dyspnea of cardiac origin. The dyspnea increases as the intensity of the cause increases. For example, an increase of blood pressure or the appearance of paroxysms of atrial fibrillation or onset of angina pectoris usually cause an increase in dyspnea. When shortness of breath increases, a cough is added, first dry, then with foamy sputum and blood. This may occur during a period of inadequate physical activity of the patient. If shortness of breath manifests at rest, then there is more accurate sign of heart failure: shortness of breath becomes heavier in a horizontal position and is relieved when the head end of the trunk is raised. The patient's forced sitting position is called orthopnea. The analysis of these features of dyspnea allows for more accurate diagnosis of heart failure.

Bendopnea, described in recent years [7], is the occurrence of shortness of breath after bending the patient sitting in a chair and pressing the abdominal belt. Shortness of breath in a patient with CHF persists for at least 30 seconds. However, this sign is not specific enough and can be observed in lung diseases and obesity [8].

Another sign of heart failure is rapid fatigue during physical activity and longer recovery after exercise. Fatigue is observed in about 85% of patients with HF [9]. The appearance of this symptom is associated with a violation of nutrition and structural adjustment of muscle tissue in patients, but may be due to hypovolemia and hypokalemia due to the use of diuretics. The specificity of the sign is extremely low, but good performance quite accurately indicates the absence of heart failure in the patient. Weakness in heart failure cannot be reduced by short-term training. In the initial stages of the disease, the patient does not feel weak at rest. It occurs only during physical activity. The patient is able to withstand short-term quite intense physical activity and at the same time gets very tired with low-intensity, but prolonged exercise. But even with these features, fatigue is a low-specific sign of heart failure.

The appearance of heaviness in the right hypochondrium indicates an increase in the liver due to stagnation in the large circle of blood circulation. The widespread pathology of the gallbladder makes this clinical sign very non-specific.

Oedema in patients with heart failure starts from the lower part of the legs and gradually involves the upper parts. In bedridden patients, edema forms on the sacrum. Oedema has a dense consistency. Their prolonged existence leads to hyperpigmentation of the skin and trophic changes in the area of oedema.

The patient's complaints must be coordinated with the physical examination data. Low exercise tolerance should correlate with the appearance of signs of congestion. The process of congestion, as a rule, from the beginning involves a small circle of blood, and for a long time during auscultation of the lungs we do not find wheezing. As a rule, wheezing in the lungs appears when the patient has shortness of breath at rest or with minimal physical activity. With long-term heart failure, a patient with wheezing lungs may not have shortness of breath at rest. Wheezing appears from the lower parts of the lungs. They are moist, small-bubbly, in the beginning not sound, but with the appearance of fibrosis of the lungs they become resounding and do not respond to treatment with diuretics.

The formation of congestion in a large circle of blood circulation is manifested by an increase and soreness of the liver. When pressing on the liver during deep breathing of the patient, you can see an increase in blood filling of the neck veins by >3 cm sustained during 10 s (hepatojugular reflux), with an abrupt fall after the pressure is released [10]. This proves the connection between an enlarged liver and increased pressure in the veins of the large circle of blood. The appearance of tricuspid insufficiency is accompanied by the occurrence of pulsation of the neck veins. Due to the decline in the contractility of the right ventricle, the patient has a decrease in shortness of breath, but an increase in weakness.

Oedema of the lower extremities sometimes precedes the appearance of hepatomegaly, but it also happens the other way around. This depends only on the innate predisposition to leg swelling and also from the patient's position. Oedema is dense in consistency, appearing first in the lower areas, then rising to the top. With long-term oedema in the area of their localization, skin atrophy occurs, hyperpigmentation appears, and the skin becomes easily vulnerable.

The third heart tone occurs when the pressure of filling the left ventricle in the diastole is increased. Listening to the third heart tone is specific for heart failure, but it is extremely rare among outpatients.

If there is a suspicion of heart failure in the patient, you need to go upstream. In other words, it is necessary to determine the probability of developing heart failure in the patient. When communicating with the patient, you need to pay attention to the coincidence of manifestations of heart disease and possible manifestations of heart failure. In addition, it is important to determine the dependence of manifestations on heart disease. Frequent provocateurs of heart failure are uncontrolled arterial hypertension, paroxysms of fibrillation or atrial flutter, the development of acute coronary syndrome, alcohol abuse, sodium or fluid overload and the addition of infection.

To sum up, it should be noted that the accuracy of the diagnosis of HF based on clinical manifestations and physical examination data depends on the number of detected signs and symptoms, as well as on the chronological relationship with the cause of occurrence. Data analysis requires the use of clinical thinking.

5. Issues of differential diagnosis of signs and symptoms of HF

To begin differential diagnosis of manifestations similar to SN, you should always ask whether there is a reason for its development and whether the patient has a disease that can explain the manifestations. For example, if a patient has atrial fibrillation, the occurrence of shortness of breath after the development of a rhythm disorder should be explained by heart failure. And if a patient without heart disease has anemia, then shortness of breath is probably due to this cause.

But it is not necessary for a patient with heart disease to have shortness of breath only of cardiac origin. It should be mentioned once again that in every third case among outpatient visitors, who had a cardiovascular disease, HF is falsely diagnosed. And among women, this is 2 times more common than among men.

We found that most of the patients with cardiovascular disease and misdiagnosed heart failure suffer from anxiety disorders (53%). Second place is taken by obesity (39%). Then among the causes are decrepitude, pathologies of the respiratory system and anemia. There is no doubt that the patient may have different causes of symptoms.

For example, a patient with arterial hypertension and obesity may have severe anxiety and lack of training. Such a patient has a pathological circle, when anxiety for their health leads to the fact that they move less and eat more, and the increasing weight further restricts their physical abilities. These patients often have shortness of breath, oedema, enlarged liver, and arterial hypertension as a possible cause of HF. In addition, their EF remains normal, and NT-proBNP increases slightly even in the presence of HF. The cause of edema in them may be a violation of venous outflow due to obesity, or, perhaps, taking calcium antagonists, hepatomegaly is caused by non-alcoholic steatohepatitis, and shortness of breath is associated with a large body weight and lack of training.

Outpatient patients with heart failure usually have several comorbidities. So, on average, there are an additional 2.5 diseases per patient with HF. It should be noted that anxiety and depression are frequent companions of patients with HF. According to our data, 22% of outpatient patients with HF have depression, and 53% have severe anxiety.

It is necessary to distinguish between dyspnea that occurs with myocardial ischemia and dyspnea caused by HF, because dyspnea caused by ischemia is treated by restoring myocardial nutrition, and dyspnea in HF requires treatment of HF itself. If there are reasonable suspicions of an ischemic origin of dyspnea, then CT-coronary angiography should be performed.

How, then, can we distinguish HF from other causes of symptoms? To do this, you need to start treating the identified suspected cause of symptoms and evaluate the dynamics. In any case, this should be done, because if we only deal with HF without correcting comorbidities, we will not get a good clinical dynamic. But if the symptoms were associated only with extra-cardiac pathology, then we will get a brilliant result without the use of medications for HF.

6. Controversies in the use of natriuretic peptides for the verification of HF

It is known that in HF, an increase in the level of natriuretic peptides is observed in the blood. They are natural antagonists of the renin-angiotensin-aldosterone system. This is a weapon with which the patient's body resists the onslaught of neurohumoral activity in HF. However, it is very difficult to interpret the increase in the activity of these substances in a patient 2–3 times in comparison with the upper limit of the norm.

Thus, the level of brain natriuretic peptide (BNP) in obese patients is one and a half times lower compared to people with normal body weight despite a similar severity of HF [11]. In patients with liver cirrhosis, N-terminal precursor of brain natriuretic peptide (NT-proBNP) plasma level may increase five times in comparison with the control [12]. In patients with renal insufficiency, standards for the content of NT-proBNP have been developed depending on age [13].

The Association between NT-proBNP and the probability of developing atrial fibrillation [14] can be interpreted as an increase in the level of NT-proBNP in patients after silent paroxysms of atrial fibrillation. That is, the NT-proBNP level will indicate that the patient has suffered acute cardiac dysfunction, and not the presence of HF.

Thus, the abundance of parameters that affect the concentration of NT-proBNP does not allow us to make a decision about the presence or absence of HF with a small increase in its level. NTproBNP provided a higher negative predictive values (0.97) than BNP (0.87), but at lower positive predictive values (0.44 versus 0.59) [15].

In summary, it can be argued that the absence of an increase in NTproBNP can be used to exclude the diagnosis of HF, but an increase within 3 HGN should be interpreted very carefully.

Soluble ST2 receptor is a marker of the severity of fibrosis, remodeling, inflammation, and volume load on the heart. It can claim to be a more accurate marker of CH dynamics in comparison with NTproBNP [16].

On the other hand, the practitioner does not need a predictor of the developing deterioration of the patient's condition. The dynamics of body weight indicates an occurring fluid retention and the need to increase the dose of diuretics and search for the cause. And life-saving medications, such as renin-angiotensin-aldosterone system blockers, should be given at targeted doses that are independent of such markers.

7. Instrumental methods for diagnosing HF

Echocardiography is most important for confirming the diagnosis of HF as a screening method, since if EF ≤40%, the diagnosis can be considered proven. But there are few such patients in outpatient practice. Thus, most outpatient patients have diastolic heart failure. The diastolic insufficiency is the inability of the heart to accept all the blood that flows to it, while there is stagnation (increased pressure) in front of the heart chambers. This situation can occur only with physical activity, and in advanced cases also at rest.

Global longitudinal strain (GLS) is a more reproducible parameter regardless of echocardiographic training and image quality compared to EF [17]. As GLS ordinarily varies with age, sex, and LV loading conditions, defining abnormal GLS is not uncomplicated. However, in adults, GLS <16% is abnormal, GLS >18% is normal, and GLS 16–18% is borderline [18].

Traditionally, diastolic insufficiency is assessed by the ratio of the velocity of early transmitral filling (e) and the average early velocity of diastolic movement of the base of the mitral valve ring (e') [19]. It is an accurate, reliable and easily reproducible method for evaluating left ventricular diastolic function. This method does not require a sinus rhythm. In normal persons the E/e' ratio is <8. Values >14 have high specificity for increased LV filling pressures. In the range e/e' from 8 to 14, it is not possible to determine definitely the presence of HF. The accuracy of the indicator is reduced in severe mitral valve calcification, mitral valve defects, pericarditis and the presence of violations of regional contractility of the left ventricle.

Since the left atrium is also overloaded when the filling pressure of the left ventricle increases, it is important to detect the enlargement of the left atrium for the diagnosis of HF. However, it should be taken into account that the atrium can be expanded in athletes and with atrial fibrillation and flutter.

In symptomatic patients with normal levels of NTproBNP, no reduction in EF and signs of stagnation, as well as normal cardiac filling pressures at rest may have markedly abnormal hemodynamic responses during exercise [20]. An exercise pulmonary artery systolic pressure ≥ 45 mm Hg identified HF with 96% sensitivity and 95% specificity. However, such invasive tests are not acceptable for outpatient clinics.

If the etiology of HF is unclear, the need to assess the structures of the heart and surrounding tissues, assess the severity of fibrosis, differential diagnosis of inflammatory, accumulative and ischemic causes, the patient should perform cardiovascular magnetic resonance (CMR) tracking with or without an assessment of late gadolinium enhancement (LGE). A fast long-axis strain (FLAS) at end-systole of 12.3% and less predict the presence of HF [21]. The sensitivity and specificity of the method is 93% and 86%, respectively. This method is reproducible, reliable, and effective, but expensive.

8. Use of acute medication tests for the diagnosis of HF

It is known that the manifestation of congestion is best reversed against the background of the use of diuretics, while congestion in the lungs is quickly stopped by nitroglycerin. However, nitroglycerin is poorly tolerated by some patients, and it can also be effective for spasms of any origin, including bronchial asthma. Thus, the specificity of reducing shortness of breath after using nitroglycerin is not great. The use of diuretics seems to be a more effective way to detect the relationship of low exercise tolerance with fluid retention in the patient's body.

A sample with torasemide was developed for use in outpatient clinics for the differential diagnosis of dyspnea of cardiac and non-cardiac origin with a sensitivity of 89% and specificity of 82%.

Method of performing the test [22]. In the morning, all patients undergo a 6-minute walking test. Then the patient should take torasemide 5 mg. 6-minute walking test is repeated every other day, all other things being equal. The increase in walking distance should be at least 15 m.

The test with torasemide is not expensive and can be performed by any medical professional without special training. The test can be used as the first stage of differential diagnosis in an outpatient environment in a patient with cardiovascular disease and dyspnea of unknown origin.

9. Complex systems for assessing the probability of having HF

The newly created H2FPEF score allows you to accurately and quickly assess the probability of having HF in a patient [23]. Obesity (body mass index >30 kg/m^2), atrial fibrillation, age > 60 years, treatment with ≥2 antihypertensive drugs, E/e' > 9, and pulmonary artery systolic pressure > 35 mm Hg were associated with HF. Atrial fibrillation gives 3 points, obesity - 2 points, other signs-1 point each. If the scale value is 0–1, it is very likely to exclude SN, if it is 6 or more points, it confirms it. Values from 2 to 5 require the use of clarifying methods (**Figure 1**).

The 'HFA-PEFF diagnostic algorithm' is also proposed [24]. In accordance with this algorithm, a pre-test assessment of the probability of CH is first performed. For this purpose, the presence of such risk factors for HF as obesity, hypertension, diabetes mellitus, the elderly, and atrial fibrillation is evaluated. Routine laboratory tests (sodium, potassium, urea, and creatinine, liver function tests, HbA1c, thyroid stimulating hormone, full blood count, ferritin, transferrin saturation, and hemoglobin), electrocardiogram and echocardiography are performed. In the absence of an obvious extracardial cause of symptoms and the presence of risk factors for heart failure, even at normal levels of natriuretic peptides, HF should be suspected.

The next step is an in-depth echocardiographic study, including E/e', left atrial volume index, LV mass index, relative LV wall thickness, tricuspid regurgitation rate, global longitudinal LV systolic strain, and serum natriuretic peptide levels if not already done (**Table 1**). If the sum of points of the HFA–PEFF Score is 1 and less than points, the diagnosis of CH is considered unlikely, if 5 the diagnosis of CH is proven. Sum 2–4 requires a transition to the next stage of diagnostics.

At Step 3 is recommended an echocardiographic or invasive hemodynamic exercise stress tests. The HF criteria for performing stress echocardiography are the average E/e 'ratio at peak stress increases to ≥15, with or without a peak tricuspid regurgitation velocity of >3.4 m/s. If the above-mentioned signs are not detected during the exercise echocardiography, then an invasive test should have performed. An elevated LV filling pressures at rest (LVEDP ≥16 mmHg) or/and a high mean pulmonary capillary wedge pressure (mPCWP≥15 mmHg) at rest is confirmed HF.

	Clinical Variable	Values	Points
H_2	Heavy	Body mass index > 30 kg/m²	2
	Hypertensive	2 or more antihypertensive medicines	1
F	Atrial Fibrillation	Paroxysmal or Persistent	3
P	Pulmonary Hypertension	Doppler Echocardiographic estimated Pulmonary Artery Systolic Pressure > 35 mmHg	1
E	Elder	Age > 60 years	1
F	Filling Pressure	Doppler Echocardiographic E/e' > 9	1
	H_2FPEF score		Sum (0-9)

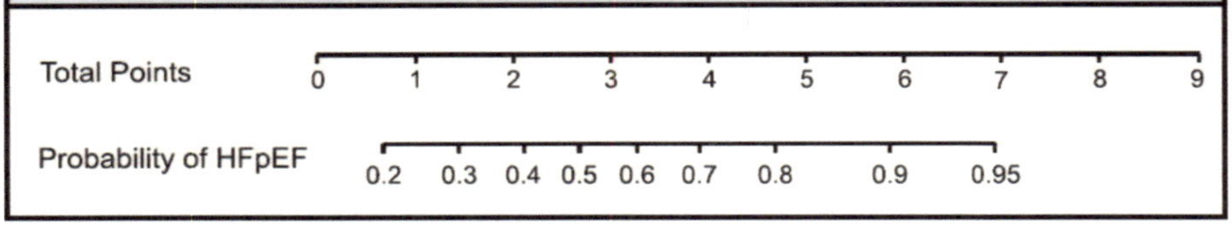

Figure 1.
The H2FPEF score with associated probability of having heart failure [23].

Measurement	Criterion	Points
A. Functional Measurement Domain		
e'	Age < 75 years:	
Peak early diastolic velocity of mitral annular motion (cm/s)	Septal e' < 7 or lateral e' < 10	2
	Age ≥ 75 years:	
	Septal e' < 5 or lateral e' < 7	2
E/e' as major criterion		
Peak early diastolic velocity of mitral inflow, divided by the mean value of e' recorded at the septal and lateral mitral annulus	E/e' ratio ≥ 15	2
Tricuspid regurgitation velocity (m/s)	Peak velocity > 2.8	2
E/e' as minor criterion	E/e' ratio 9–14	1
Global longitudinal strain (GLS) of the LV in systole (%, as positive value)	GLS < 16	1
B. Morphological Measurement Domain		
Left atrial volume index (ml/m2) as major criterion	Patient in sinus rhythm:	
	> 34	2
	Patient in atrial fibrillation: > 40	2
Left ventricular hypertrophy (major)		
LV mass index (LVMI) in g/m²	Male patient:	
LV relative wall thickness (RWT)	LVMI ≥149 and RWT > 0.42	2
	Female patient:	

Measurement	Criterion	Points
	LVMI ≥122 and RWT > 0.42	2
Left atrial volume index (ml/m2) as minor criterion	Patient in sinus rhythm:	
	29–34	1
	Patient in atrial fibrillation:	
	34–40	1
Left ventricular hypertrophy	Male patient:	
Minor criteria:	LVMI ≥115	
LV mass index (LVMI) in g/m2	RWT > 0.42	
LV relative wall thickness (RWT)	LV wall thickness ≥ 12	
LV wall thickness (mm)	Any 1 criterion positive	1
	2 or 3 positive	1
	Female patient:	
	LVMI ≥95	
	RWT > 0.42	
	LV wall thickness ≥ 12	
	Any 1 criterion positive	1
	2 or 3 positive	1
C. Natriuretic Peptide Domain		
Serum concentration of brain natriuretic peptide (BNP) or N-terminal proBNP (NT-proBNP) (pg/ml or ng/L)	Patient in sinus rhythm:	
	BNP > 80	2
	BNP 35–80	1
	NT-proBNP >220	2
	NT-proBNP 125–220	1
	Patient in atrial fibrillation:	
	BNP > 240	2
	BNP 105–240	1
	NT-proBNP >660	2
	NT-proBNP 375–660	1
From 0 to maximal 2 points per domain		
Select only 1 score from each domain (A, B, C) TOTAL		
Unlikely ≤1		
Intermediate 2–4		
Probable ≥5		

Table 1.
The HFA–PEFF score (step 2).

In the absence of detection of these indicators, a stress test is required. An increase in peak exercise PCWP ≥25 mmHg is interpreted as proof of the diagnosis of HF.

Step 4 involves clarifying the cause of HF. Sometimes it is necessary to perform cardiac magnetic resonance imaging, computed tomography, positron emission tomography, myocardial biopsy, genetic and special laboratory tests.

Performing the algorithm further in step 2 is not appropriate for routine practice due to the need for high-level specialists and the need for invasive diagnostics, which increases the risk for the patient. Moreover, difficulties may arise even when evaluating E/e' [25].

10. Conclusions

The diagnosis of HF in an outpatient setting is a difficult task. First, it is necessary to determine the clinical probability of HF by the features of manifestations, their dynamics, and risk factors. Then, to clarify the presence of diseases that could explain the symptoms, to assess the EF. In the absence of a reduction in EF ≤40%, it is required to calculate the HFA-PEFF Score (a more complex and expensive variant) or H2FPEF score (a cheaper and more available option, but less precise). If tissue Doppler imaging is not available, a torasemide test should be used for differential diagnosis of dyspnea.

In any case, it is impossible to allow the risk of performing a patient's examination to exceed the benefit of the information received. The examination should be sufficient to make an adequate decision about the treatment of the patient, and not be the goal itself.

Acknowledgements

The writing of this chapter was not financially supported.

Conflict of interest

The authors declare no conflict of interest.

Thanks

We thank our mentor Professor Leonid Polikarpov for his kindness and pointing out the right path.

Author details

Oleg Anatolievich Shtegman* and Marina Mihailovna Petrova
Federal State Budgetary Educational Institution of Higher Education "Krasnoyarsk State Medical University Named after Professor V.F. Vojno-Yasenetsky" of the Ministry of Health of the Russian Federation, Krasnoyarsk, Russia

*Address all correspondence to: cvb2@list.ru

References

[1] Groenewegen A, Rutten FH, Mosterd A, Hoes AW. Epidemiology of heart failure. Eur J Heart Fail. 2020;22(8):1342-1356. DOI: 10.1002/ejhf.1858

[2] Trullàs JC, Casado J, Morales-Rull JL. Difficulties in the diagnosis of heart failure in patients with comorbidities. Rev Clin Esp. 2016;216(5):276-85. English, Spanish. DOI: 10.1016/j.rce.2015.10.001

[3] Mareev VJu, Danieljan MO, Belenkov JuN. Comparative characteristics of patients with CHF, depending on the size of the ejection fraction by the results of the Russian multicenter study AGE-O-CHF: again about the problem of heart failure with preserved left ventricular systolic function. Serdechnaya nedostatochnost. 2006; 4: 164-71. Russian DOI: 10.18087/rhfj2015.1.2038.

[4] Petrova M.M., Shtegman O.A., Chernykh P.V., Kovaltsova K.A. Prevalence of chronic heart failure in ambulatory practice in Krasnoyarsk. Modern Problems of Science and Education. 2011;3; URL: http://science-education.ru/ru/article/view?id=4671 (date of request: 15.11.2020)

[5] Owan TE, Hodge DO, Herges RM, Jacobsen SJ, Roger VL, Redfield MM. Trends in prevalence and outcome of heart failure with preserved ejection fraction. N Engl J Med. 2006 Jul 20;355(3):251-9. DOI: 10.1056/NEJMoa052256.

[6] Davie AP, Francis CM, Caruana L, Sutherland GR, McMurray JJ. Assessing diagnosis in heart failure: which features are any use?. QJM. 1997; 90:335-9.

[7] Thibodeau JT, Turer AT, Gualano SK, Ayers CR, Velez-Martinez M, Mishkin JD, Patel PC, Mammen PP, Markham DW, Levine BD, Drazner MH. Characterization of a novel symptom of advanced heart failure: bendopnea. JACC Heart Fail. 2014;2(1):24-31. DOI: 10.1016/j.jchf.2013.07.009

[8] Thibodeau JT, Drazner MH. The Role of the Clinical Examination in Patients With Heart Failure. JACC Heart Fail. 2018;6(7):543-551. DOI: 10.1016/j.jchf.2018.04.005

[9] Alpert CM, Smith MA, Hummel SL, Hummel EK. Symptom burden in heart failure: assessment, impact on outcomes, and management. Heart Fail Rev. 2017;22(1):25-39. DOI: 10.1007/s10741-016-9581-4.

[10] Ducas J, Magder S, McGregor M. Validity of the hepatojugular reflux as a clinical test for congestive heart failure. Am J Cardiol. 1983 Dec 1;52(10):1299-303. DOI: 10.1016/0002-9149(83)90592-1

[11] Mehra MR, Uber PA, Park MH, Scott RL, Ventura HO, Harris BC, Frohlich ED. Obesity and suppressed B-type natriuretic peptide levels in heart failure. J Am Coll Cardiol. 2004;43(9):1590-5. DOI: 10.1016/j.jacc.2003.10.066. PMID: 15120816.

[12] Licata A, Corrao S, Petta S, Genco C, Cardillo M, Calvaruso V, Cabibbo G, Massenti F, Cammà C, Licata G, Craxì A. NT pro BNP plasma level and atrial volume are linked to the severity of liver cirrhosis. PLoS One. 2013;8(8):e68364. DOI: 10.1371/journal.pone.0068364

[13] DeFilippi C, van Kimmenade RR, Pinto YM. Amino-terminal pro-B-type natriuretic peptide testing in renal disease. Am J Cardiol. 2008;101(3A):82-8. DOI: 10.1016/j.amjcard.2007.11.029.

[14] Li L, Selvin E, Lutsey PL, Hoogeveen RC, O'Neal WT, Soliman EZ, Chen LY, Alonso A.

Association of N-terminal pro B-type natriuretic peptide (NT-proBNP) change with the risk of atrial fibrillation in the ARIC cohort. Am Heart J. 2018;204:119-127. DOI: 10.1016/j.ahj.2018.07.008

[15] Zaphiriou A, Robb S, Murray-Thomas T, Mendez G, Fox K, McDonagh T, Hardman SM, Dargie HJ, Cowie MR. The diagnostic accuracy of plasma BNP and NTproBNP in patients referred from primary care with suspected heart failure: results of the UK natriuretic peptide study. Eur J Heart Fail. 2005;7(4):537-41. DOI: 10.1016/j.ejheart.2005.01.022

[16] Van Vark LC, Lesman-Leegte I, Baart SJ, Postmus D, Pinto YM, Orsel JG et al. Prognostic Value of Serial ST2 Measurements in Patients with Acute Heart Failure. Journal of the American College of Cardiology. 2017;70(19):2378-88. DOI: 10.1016/j.jacc.2017.09.026

[17] Karlsen S, Dahlslett T, Grenne B, Sjøli B, Smiseth O, Edvardsen T, Brunvand H. Global longitudinal strain is a more reproducible measure of left ventricular function than ejection fraction regardless of echocardiographic training. Cardiovasc Ultrasound. 2019;17(1):18. DOI: 10.1186/s12947-019-0168-9

[18] Yang H, Wright L, Negishi T, Negishi K, Liu J, Marwick TH. Research to Practice: Assessment of Left Ventricular Global Longitudinal Strain for Surveillance of Cancer Chemotherapeutic-Related Cardiac Dysfunction. JACC Cardiovasc Imaging. 2018 Aug;11(8):1196-1201. DOI: 10.1016/j.jcmg.2018.07.005

[19] Nagueh SF, Smiseth OA, Appleton CP, Byrd BF 3rd, Dokainish H, Edvardsen T, Flachskampf FA, Gillebert TC, Klein AL, Lancellotti P, Marino P, Oh JK, Popescu BA, Waggoner AD. Recommendations for the Evaluation of Left Ventricular Diastolic Function by Echocardiography: An Update from the American Society of Echocardiography and the European Association of Cardiovascular Imaging. J Am Soc Echocardiogr. 2016 Apr;29(4):277-314. DOI: 10.1016/j.echo.2016.01.011

[20] Borlaug BA, Nishimura RA, Sorajja P, Lam CS, Redfield MM. Exercise hemodynamics enhance diagnosis of early heart failure with preserved ejection fraction. Circ Heart Fail. 2010;3(5):588-95. DOI: 10.1161/CIRCHEARTFAILURE.109.930701

[21] Leng S, Tan RS, Zhao X, Allen JC, Koh AS, Zhong L. Fast long-axis strain: a simple, automatic approach for assessing left ventricular longitudinal function with cine cardiovascular magnetic resonance. Eur Radiol. 2020 Jul;30(7):3672-3683. DOI: 10.1007/s00330-020-06744-6

[22] Shtegman OA, Shiriaev IV, Frolkina MO. Test with torasemide in the differential diagnosis of dyspnea in patients with cardiovascular diseases. Kardiologiia. 2014;54(11):30-3. Russian. DOI: 10.18565/cardio.2014.11.30-33

[23] Reddy YNV, Carter RE, Obokata M, Redfield MM, Borlaug BA. A Simple, Evidence-Based Approach to Help Guide Diagnosis of Heart Failure With Preserved Ejection Fraction. Circulation. 2018 Aug 28;138(9):861-870. DOI: 10.1161/CIRCULATIONAHA.118.034646

[24] Pieske B, Tschöpe C, de Boer RA, Fraser AG, Anker SD, Donal E, Edelmann F, Fu M, Guazzi M, Lam CSP, Lancellotti P, Melenovsky V, Morris DA, Nagel E, Pieske-Kraigher E, Ponikowski P, Solomon SD, Vasan RS, Rutten FH, Voors AA, Ruschitzka F, Paulus WJ, Seferovic P, Filippatos G. How to diagnose heart failure with preserved ejection fraction: the HFA-PEFF diagnostic algorithm: a consensus

recommendation from the Heart Failure Association (HFA) of the European Society of Cardiology (ESC). Eur J Heart Fail. 2020 Mar;22(3):391-412. DOI: 10.1002/ejhf.1741.

[25] Obokata M, Borlaug BA. The strengths and limitations of E/e' in heart failure with preserved ejection fraction. Eur J Heart Fail. 2018 Sep;20(9):1312-1314. DOI: 10.1002/ejhf.1250

Chapter 5

Advances in Outpatient Hysteroscopy

Ayesha Ajmi

Abstract

Hysteroscopy is a gynaecological procedure that has developed into an important tool to identify endometrial abnormality. It offers direct examination of the uterine cavity and tubal ostia and offers the option of performing targeted biopsy of suspected lesions that can be missed by blind procedures. In a large number of cases, the intrauterine lesions can be diagnosed and treated at the same setting as one step approach ("see and treat"). For example, endometrial polyps can be identified and removed; intrauterine adhesions may be divided in the office owing to the practicability of operative saline hysteroscopy, vaginoscopic approach and the convenience of miniature hysteroscopes. There is decent evidence that hysteroscopy in the outpatient clinic setting is preferred by the patients, associated with low risk of complications, quicker recovery time and reduced cost. Technological advances have led to development of high definition miniature hysteroscopes without negotiating optical performance, and hence making hysteroscopy an ingenuous, safe and trusted office procedure. Recent advances such as bipolar electrosurgery, endometrial ablation devices, morcellators and tissue retrieval system has transformed the surgical technique. This modernization of hysteroscopy completely revolutionised the approach to the management of intrauterine pathologies, moving from a blind procedure under general anaesthesia to directly visualised procedure under no or local anaesthesia, offering diagnostic as well as therapeutic procedures that should be at the disposal of every modern gynaecologist.

Keywords: outpatient hysteroscopy, office hysteroscopy, ambulatory hysteroscopy, vaginoscopy, polypectomy

1. Introduction

Hysteroscopy represents the endoscopic gynaecological examination of the endometrial cavity and denotes one of the most frequent investigations in gynaecology today, used in the diagnostic work up of abnormal uterine bleeding, postmenopausal bleeding and subfertility. The National Institute for Health and Care Excellence recommends an enhanced role of outpatient hysteroscopy in the diagnostic workup of heavy menstrual bleeding, leading to increase in the number of hysteroscopies being performed each year [1, 2]. Abnormal uterine bleeding in both the premenopausal and postmenopausal women is the commonest indication for diagnostic hysteroscopy. Similarly endometrial polyp is the most frequent preoperative indication for operative hysteroscopy followed by submucosal leiomyoma [3]. In a retrospective clinical study of 397 patients, dilatation and curettage failed to identify pathology in 62.5% cases subsequently found at hysterectomy within

2 months [4]. A large clinical observational study demonstrated that up to 3.7 cm pathology could be safely treated by office hysteroscopy without anaesthesia [5]. Paracervical block is however commonly used for operative hysteroscopy where cervical dilatation is required [6].

During hysteroscopy it is recommended to provide the patient with emotional support ("local-vocal"), by chatting to her and offering her to look at the monitor while explaining the findings to her in order to avoid feeling of exclusion. Dedicated nursing and healthcare assistant staff is crucial in ambulatory setting. It is recommended for patients to take 400 mg of ibuprofen or another NSAID approximately 1 hour before the procedure.

2. Vaginoscopy

The traditional approach to hysteroscopy is by utilising a vaginal speculum with or without manipulation of the cervix.

Vaginoscopy refers to a method where the hysteroscope is guided into the uterus without having to use the potentially painful vaginal instruments. The availability of miniature hysteroscopes has facilitated this development. A randomised controlled multicentre trial in the UK concluded that vaginoscopy is quicker to perform, less painful, and more successful than standard hysteroscopy and therefore should be regarded as the technique of choice for outpatient hysteroscopy [7, 8].

3. Outpatient diagnostic hysteroscopy

3.1 Abnormal uterine bleeding (AUB) in women of reproductive age group

The hysteroscopy has been gold standard in the examination of the endometrial cavity in ladies with abnormal uterine bleeding for several years. In the UK, the national best practice recommendation is that all gynaecology departments should offer dedicated outpatient hysteroscopy facility to support the diagnosis and treatment of ladies with abnormal uterine bleeding. The advances in outpatient hysteroscopy have further powered the use of this facility, and it is not required any more to put patients through general anaesthesia for this purpose [9]. In most women, the diagnosis for abnormal uterine bleeding can be made in the outpatient clinic with one-stop approach with a host of other investigations, including blood tests, pelvic ultrasound, outpatient hysteroscopy and endometrial biopsy. The prompt diagnosis permits timely treatment, avoiding unnecessary delays and patient anxiety [10].

A large number of women presenting with AUB belong to the reproductive age group. The causative factors may be structural abnormalities such as endometrial polyps or fibroids or ovulatory dysfunction and primary disorder of endometrium as described in the PALM-COEIN classification (**Figure 1**). These abnormalities can be readily diagnosed in outpatient setting by ambulatory hysteroscopy with or without endometrial biopsy [11–13]. **Figure 2** shows office hysteroscope with different channels for diagnosis as well as removal of pathology.

3.2 Perimenopausal bleeding

For women in this age group presenting with new onset abnormal uterine bleeding, organic pathology, such as atypical hyperplasia or endometrial cancer, must be ruled out as anovulatory cycles and sinister pathology can coexist, in this cohort of women (**Figure 3**).

DOI: http://dx.doi.org/10.5772/intechopen.97093

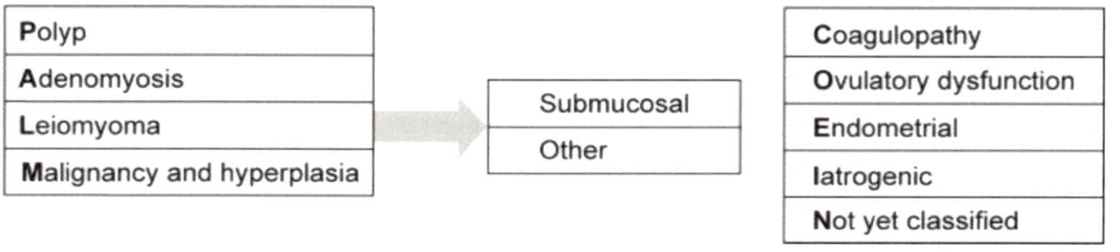

Figure 1.
FIGO classification of PALM-COEIN system. Abbreviation: FIGO, International Federation of Gynaecology and Obstetrics.

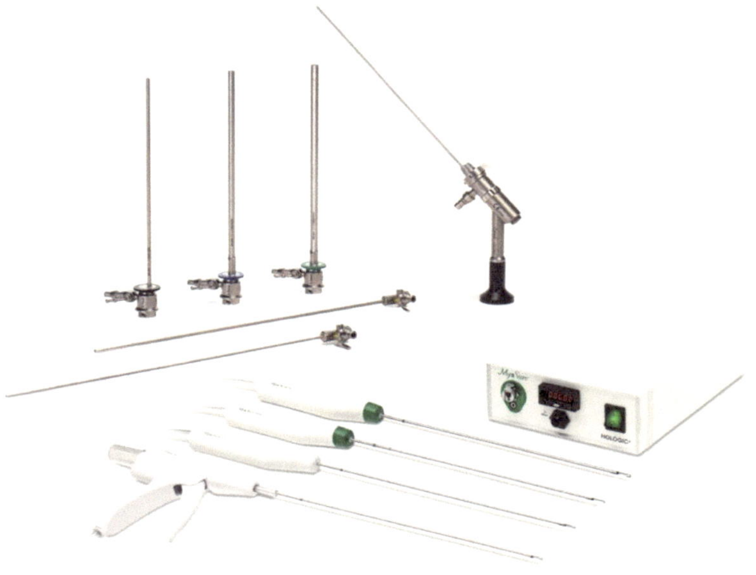

Figure 2.
Omni-myosure (HOLOGIC).

Endorsed pelvic ultrasound scan as the first-line tool for identifying structural abnormalities. Hysteroscopy remains the gold standard for precise evaluation of endometrial cavity. Indications for endometrial biopsy include women ≥45 years of age, failed or ineffective treatment, persistent intermenstrual bleeding and co-existence of risk factors demonstrated in **Figure 2**.

3.3 Postmenopausal bleeding

Hysteroscopy is established as the gold standard in the evaluation of AUB in postmenopausal women, eliminating the false-negative results of blind biopsy by direct visualisation of the endometrial cavity and enabling targeted biopsy if warranted [14]. It allows full visualisation of the endocervix, endometrial cavity and tubal ostia, permitting diagnosis of endometrial lesions that may be missed with blind endometrial sampling, TVS or even saline infusion sonography (SIS). Moreover, vaginoscopic technique to perform office hysteroscopy can also be employed for careful examination of possible vaginal and cervical lesion that may be responsible for abnormal uterine bleeding. This approach also reduces discomfort in women, including virgins, older women and those with moderate stenosis of the cervical os who would have required general anaesthesia otherwise.

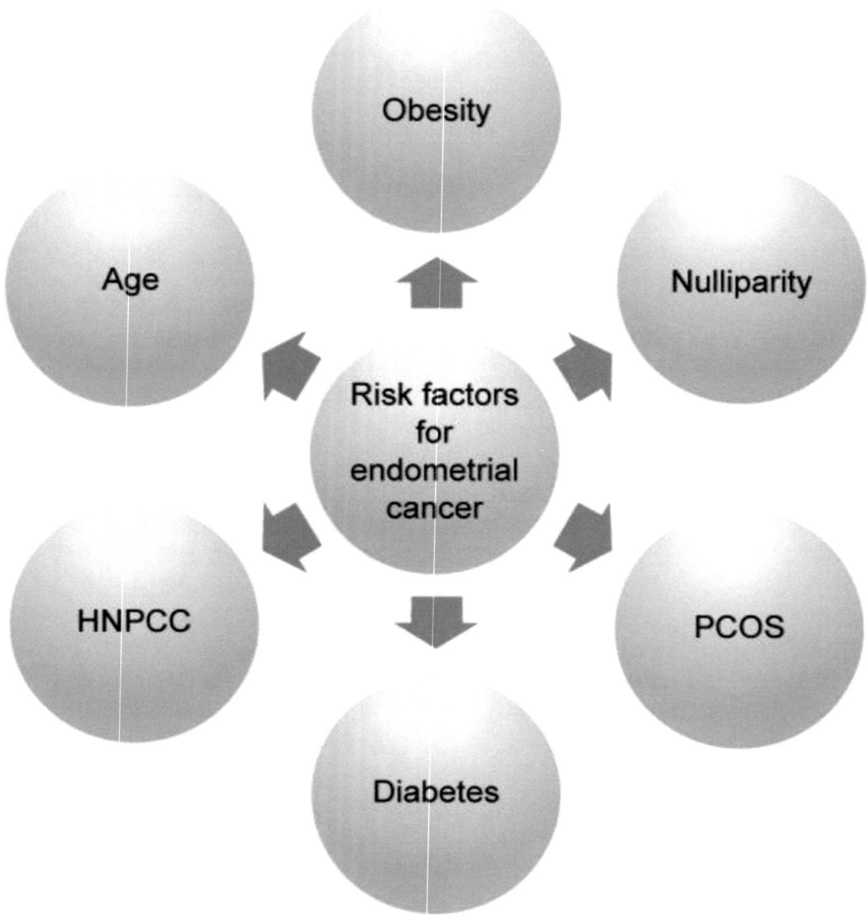

Figure 3.
Risk factors for endometrial cancer. Abbreviations: PCOS, polycystic ovarian syndrome; HNPCC, hereditary non-polyposis colorectal cancer.

The sensitivity, specificity and high precision of hysteroscopy are well established. With miniaturisation of hysteroscopes and newer treatment techniques such as bipolar devices and hysteroscopic tissue removal systems, outpatient hysteroscopy is no longer just a diagnostic test but can offer one stop treatment to women presenting with AUB [15–17].

4. Outpatient operative hysteroscocopy

4.1 Hysteroscopic polypectomy

Uterine polyps are focal endometrial outgrowths that may appear anywhere in the uterine cavity (**Figure 4**). They comprise of a variable amount of glands, stroma and blood vessels. Endometrial polyps are commonly found in combination with AUB. They affect women of reproductive age as well as postmenopausal women. Their underlying aetiology is unsure, but most are benign. Hysteroscopy is the gold standard diagnostic test. Diagnosis at outpatient hysteroscopy allows for simultaneous surgical removal, which is convenient for most women. Polyps should

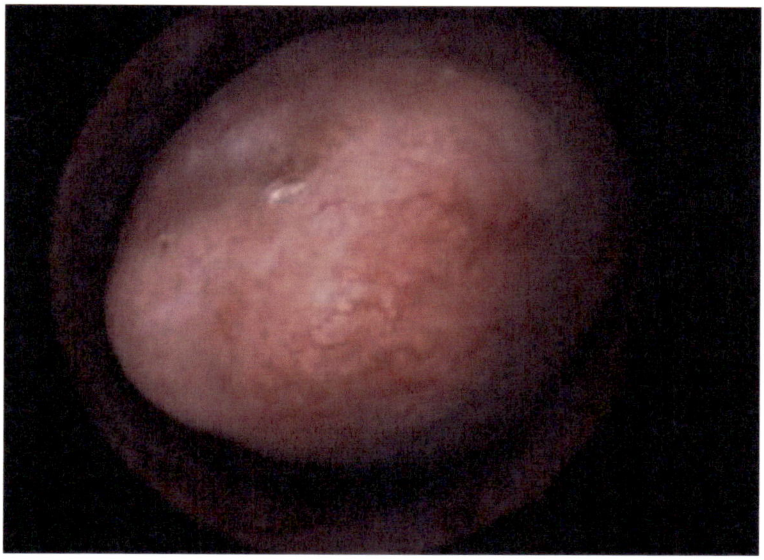

Figure 4.
Hysteroscopic appearance of an endometrial polyp.

be removed in entirety in women with post-menopausal bleeding because 6% of the polyps harbour atypical endometrial hyperplasia or cancer particularly at the base [18–21].

Video 1 https://youtu.be/HkbCZ318vJ8 outpatient hysteroscopic polypectomy procedure.

Outpatient polypectomy has been shown to be non-inferior to the inpatient procedure [22].

Uterine polypectomy could only be performed in the past using blind procedures, such as curettage and blind avulsion with forceps. To introduce such instruments required dilatation of the cervix and manipulation within the uterine cavity, that necessitated general anaesthesia. Developments in hysteroscopic equipment have enabled polyps to be removed using fine mechanical and electrosurgical tools, which are introduced down a 5- or 7-French rigid operating hysteroscope, and lately, the development of bespoke tissue removal systems. These techniques involve hysteroscopic assessment of uterine cavity, removal of the polyp from the uterine wall and retrieval using the same kit.

The enhanced fastidiousness of surgery and bypassing the requisite for routine significant cervical dilatation have empowered this to become a useful procedure, which can be performed in the office. Often local anaesthesia is not required, especially when using miniature hysteroscopes and employing vaginoscopic technique. Intracervical or paracervical injection of local anaesthesia may be used if cervical dilatation is required [23].

The results of the OPT trial exhibited that outpatient polypectomy was comparable to inpatient polypectomy for the effective mitigation of uterine bleeding due to uterine polyps. At 6 months, 73% of women in the outpatient treatment group and 80% in the inpatient treatment group were effectively cured, and the treatment effects were sustained at 12 and 24 months.

A patient preference study was conducted alongside this RCT which demonstrated a strong treatment setting preference. Nearly, 81% women in this study expressed an inclination for outpatient treatment, and a formal structured interview and thematic analysis established that the overall convenience and feasibility of the outpatient procedure, precluding hospital admission and time off work was highly valued by the women and outweighed the discomfort of the procedure [24].

4.2 Outpatient endometrial ablation

Heavy menstrual bleeding affects one in five premenopausal women and significantly impairs quality of life. There is evidence to offer endometrial ablation as a first line surgical option for the management of heavy menstrual bleeding. Hysteroscopy and endometrial biopsy should be performed prior to the procedure to rule out any organic pathology and after the procedure to rule out uterine perforation. Endometrial ablation in outpatient setting is associated with shorter hospital stay and quicker recovery. The development of newer (second generation) endometrial ablation techniques has empowered clinicians to set up a comprehensive outpatient service to treat heavy menstrual bleeding effectively without the need for general anaesthetic or conscious sedation. An observational study was performed in ladies with heavy menstrual bleeding who consented to have endometrial ablation in the outpatient setting under local anaesthetic. Once started, the ablation procedure did not have to be abandoned. Eighty-nine percent women went home immediately. Ninety percent expressed that they would have ambulatory hysteroscopic procedure if required in future. Endometrial ablation has conventionally been performed under general anaesthesia as a day case procedure. With new second-generation devices, which enable shorter treatment times, it has become more practical to perform the procedure in outpatient setting. Gynaecologists should continue to offer outpatient endometrial ablation to appropriately selected patients with abnormal uterine bleeding, with adequate counselling regarding possible pain and discomfort and alternative options [25].

Video 2 Novasure® Endometrial Ablation https://youtu.be/I2NOl9xb1os.

5. Conclusions

Hysteroscopy under direct vision can be considered as the gold standard for examination of the uterine cavity, bypassing the significant limitations and possible complications of blind procedures. Modern technological advancements have brought ambulatory hysteroscopy to a mainstay in modern gynaecological practice.

The "see & treat hysteroscopy", has revolutionised the management of abnormal uterine bleeding in all age groups. It has reduced the distinction between diagnostic and operative procedure, introducing the concept of a one step procedure perfectly amalgamating the treatment side with the diagnostic work-up. The use of miniaturised mechanical instruments together with the use of small diameter scopes with working channels and continuous flow systems, has enabled "see & treat" hysteroscopy in the office setting [26].

Outpatient hysteroscopy with direct visualisation represents the optimal diagnostic modality for abnormal uterine bleeding in premenopausal and postmenopausal women as well as treatment option for heavy menstrual bleeding, endometrial polyp, submucosal fibroid type 0 to 2, intrauterine adhesions and uterine septum. It provides cavity assessment in patients with subfertility as well [27]. Most women believe that the overall convenience of the office based procedure outweighs the pain and discomfort experienced and opt for the office procedure if required in future [28]. Hysteroscopy is generally a safe procedure and the uncommon complications such as infection, uterine perforation and fluid overload can be minimised by training, meticulous technique and modern equipment [29, 30].

Acknowledgements

Figures and videos "courtesy of HOLOGIC, Inc. and affiliates."

Conflict of interest

The author declares no conflict of interest.

Author details

Ayesha Ajmi
Bolton Foundation NHS Trust, Bolton, UK

*Address all correspondence to: ayesha.q.ajmi@gmail.com

References

[1] Heavy menstrual bleeding: assessment and management| Guidance and guidelines | NICE [Internet] [www.nice.org.uk/guidance/ng88]. Accessed 09 March 2019 Google Scholar

[2] Clark T.J., Gupta J.K.: Handbook of outpatient hysteroscopy: a complete guide to diagnosis and therapy.2005. CRC PressBoca Raton, FL

[3] Kayatas S, Meseci E, Tosun OA, Arinkan SA, Uygur L, Api M. Experience of hysteroscopy indications and complications in 5,474 cases. Clin Exp Obstet Gynecol. 2014;41(4):451-454

[4] Bettocchi S, Ceci O, Vicino M, Marello F, Impedovo L, Selvaggi L. Diagnostic inadequacy of dilatation and curettage. Fertil Steril. 2001;75(4):803-805

[5] Cicinelli E. Hysteroscopy without anesthesia: review of recent literature. J Minim Invasive Gynecol.2010;17(6):703-708.

[6] O'Flynn H, Murphy LL, Ahmad G, Watson AJ. Pain relief in outpatient hysteroscopy: a survey of current UK clinical practice. Eur J Obstet Gynecol Reprod Biol. 2011;154(1):9-15.

[7] Smith, PP, Kolhe, S, O'Connor, S, Clark, TJ. Vaginoscopy Against Standard Treatment: a randomised controlled trial. BJOG 2019; 126: 891-899.

[8] Bettocchi S, Selvaggi L. A vaginoscopic approach to reduce the pain of office hysteroscopy. J Am Assoc Gynecol Laparosc. 1997;4(2):255-258

[9] Bakour SH, Jones SE, O'Donovan P. Ambulatory hysteroscopy: evidence-based guide to diagnosis and therapy. Best Pract Res Clin Obstet Gynaecol. 2006;20(6):953-975.

[10] Bradley LD. Diagnosis of abnormal uterine bleeding with biopsy or hysteroscopy. Menopause. 2011;18(4):425-433

[11] Kolhe S. Management of abnormal uterine bleeding - focus on ambulatory hysteroscopy. Int J Womens Health. 2018 Mar 22;10:127-136. doi: 10.2147/IJWH.S98579. PMID: 29606892; PMCID: PMC5868607.

[12] Van Dongen H, de Kroon CD, Jacobi CE, Trimbos JB, Jansen FW. Diagnostic hysteroscopy in abnormal uterine bleeding: a systematic review and meta-analysis. BJOG. 2007;114(6):664-675

[13] Munro MG, Critchley HO, Broder MS, Fraser IS, FIGO Working Group on Menstrual Disorders FIGO classification system (PALM-COEIN) for causes of abnormal uterine bleeding in nongravid women of reproductive age. Int J Gynaecol Obstet. 2011;113(1):3-13. [PubMed] [Google Scholar]

[14] Cooper NA, Barton PM, Breijer M, et al. Cost-effectiveness of diagnostic strategies for the management of abnormal uterine bleeding (heavy menstrual bleeding and post-menopausal bleeding): a decision analysis. Health Technol Assess. 2014;18(24):1-201. v–vi

[15] Angioni S, Loddo A, Milano F, Piras B, Minerba L, Melis GB. Detection of benign intracavitary lesions in postmenopausal women with abnormal uterine bleeding: a prospective comparative study on outpatient hysteroscopy and blind biopsy. J Minim Invasive Gynecol. 2008;15(1):87-91. [PubMed] [Google Scholar]

[16] Grimbizis GF, Tsolakidis D, Mikos T, et al. A prospective comparison of transvaginal ultrasound, saline infusion

sonohysterography, and diagnostic hysteroscopy in the evaluation of endometrial pathology. Fertil Steril. 2010;94(7):2720-2725. [PubMed] [Google Scholar

[17] T. Justin Clark, Helen Stevenson,Endometrial Polyps and Abnormal Uterine Bleeding (AUB-P): What is the relationship, how are they diagnosed and how are they treated?,Best Practice & Research Clinical Obstetrics & Gynaecology,2017;40:89-104 ISSN 1521-6934, https://doi.org/10.1016/j.bpobgyn.2016.09.005

[18] Elfayomy A.K., Habib F.A., Alkabalawy M.A.: Role of hysteroscopy in the detection of endometrial pathologies in women presenting with postmenopausal bleeding and thickened endometrium. Arch Gynecol Obstet 2012; 285: pp. 839-843.

[19] Nathani F, Clark TJ. Uterine polypectomy in the management of abnormal uterine bleeding: a systematic review. J Minim Invasive Gynecol. 2006;13(4):260-268.

[20] Bakour S.H., Khan K.S., Gupta J.K.: The risk of premalignant and malignant pathology in endometrial polyps. Acta Obstet Gynecol Scand 2002; 8: pp. 182-183

[21] Daniele A, Ferrero A, Maggiorotto F, Perrini G, Volpi E, Sismondi P. Suspecting malignancy in endometrial polyps: value of hysteroscopy. Tumori. 2013;99(2):204-209

[22] Cooper NA, Clark TJ, Middleton L, et al. Outpatient versus inpatient uterine polyp treatment for abnormal uterine bleeding: randomised controlled non-inferiority study. BMJ. 2015;350:h1398.

[23] Garuti G., Centinaio G., Luerti M.: Outpatient hysteroscopic polypectomy in postmenopausal women: a comparison between mechanical and electrosurgical resection. J Minim Invasive Gynecol 2008; 15: pp. 595-600.

[24] Clark T.J., Middleton L.J., Cooper N.A.M., et. al.: A randomised controlled trial of outpatient versus inpatient Polyp Treatment (OPT) for abnormal uterine bleeding. Health Technol Assess 2015; 19:

[25] Ayesha Ajmi & Sangeeta Das (2020): Outpatient endometrial ablation: audit of outcomes and patient satisfaction, Journal of Obstetrics and Gynaecology, DOI: 10.1080/01443615.2019.1700945

[26] Campo R, Santangelo F, Gordts S, et al. Outpatient hysteroscopy. Facts Views Vis Obgyn. 2018;10(3):115-122.

[27] Salazar CA, Isaacson KB. Office Operative Hysteroscopy: An Update. J Minim Invasive Gynecol. 2018 Feb;25(2):199-208. doi: 10.1016/j.jmig.2017.08.009. Epub 2017 Aug 10. PMID: 28803811.

[28] De Iaco P, Marabini A, Stefanetti M, Del Vecchio C, Bovicelli L. Acceptability and pain of outpatient hysteroscopy. J Am Assoc Gynecol Laparosc. 2000;7(1):71-75.

[29] Stankova T, Ganovska A, Stoianova M, Kovachev S. Complications of diagnostic and operative hysteroscopy – review. Akush Ginekol. 2015;54(8):21-27.

[30] McGurgan PM, McIlwaine P. Complications of hysteroscopy and how to avoid them. Best Pract Res Clin Obstet Gynaecol. 2015;29(7):982-993.

Chapter 6

Medical Communication and SARS-CoV-2: Novel Approaches to Global Health Crises Communication as Called for by the W.H.O.

Jonathan de Rothewelle

Abstract

This analysis of medical comics has been conducted to respond to the WHO's call for health communication research during global health crises. This analysis uses a lens composed of the theories of semiotics, communication, and biomedical ethics, to assess the communicative value of SARS-CoV-2 comics as a form of health communication. The findings of this analysis show that medical comics could fulfil, in part, the WHO's call for more research on health communication during pandemics, suggesting that comics could be ethically and effectively used to disseminate information. The findings recommend a broader scope of the research of comics in medicine and call for standardized guidelines for their use.

Keywords: COVID-19, public health, medical communication, health humanities, discursive analysis, medical comics, patient education

1. Introduction

During the COVID-19 pandemic medical communication has been put to the test. The death toll continues to climb around the globe amidst mixed messaging and hopes for a return to *normal life*. First discovered in the Chinese city of Wuhan in 2019, COVID-19 is a disease that is a result of the SARS-CoV-2 virus. Due to mortality and infection rates, the World Health Organization designated it a global pandemic early on in its spread.

In a global health crisis, the healthcare industry and state health ministers rely on the effectual transmission of health communication. This communication must be of high quality and easily understandable. According to health crisis communication guidelines set by the WHO, communication during a pandemic is crucial. Communication must take place early on in the crisis and information must be constantly updated. The WHO also suggests that public health information disseminated during global health crises needs to be made available to those across various socioeconomic strata— that is, critical information must reach lower income populations and populations with lower literacy rates.

WHO guidelines recommend that this information be communicated jargon-free, in language that is easy to understand, and in various modalities, including the use of narrative and visuals. This research was developed to add to the body of literature that the World Health Organization calls for through its identified research gaps and recommendations for crisis communication (**Table 1**). This research presents comics as a viable option for effective and ethical communication during pandemics.

Confusion and the spread of misinformation during public health crises necessitates the exploration of new modalities of health communication. This study assesses the communicative value comics may have in clinical settings— the use of simple visuals and language is a method of health communication that may be highly effective. Information that is made personal and presented in a non-complex format may also be easier to remember.

Section	Recommendations	Summary of Findings
A1. Trust	"To build trust, risk communication interventions should link to functioning and accessible services, be transparent, timely, easy-to-understand, acknowledge uncertainty, address and engage affected populations, link to self-efficacy, and be disseminated using multiple platforms, methods and channels."	• To build trust during a pandemic, health authorities should focus on acknowledging uncertainty; creating scientific communication in an easy-to-understand manner; encouraging a dialogue; disseminating information through multiple platforms • Higher trust is linked to recommended actions being adopted • Trust may be based on perceptions rather than objective measures
A2. Communicating Uncertainty	"Communication by authorities to the public should include explicit information about uncertainties associated with risks, events and interventions, and indicate what is known and not known at a given time."	• Information provided to the public should include information about uncertainties • Information should be clear, avoid contradictions, and be presented in an easily understood manner • Information should be developed for different communities such as those of lower socioeconomic status • The manner in which a message is communicated is as important as the message content itself
B3. Capacity Building	"Preparation and training of personnel for ERC should be organized regularly and focus on coordination across involved stakeholders."	Capacities that need to be strengthened include: • Softer communication and interpersonal skills along with consensus-building • Development of communication strategies, plans and standards of practice • Translation of technical communications into understandable, contextualized material

Table 1.
Summary of World Health Organization Findings, Recommendations, and Research Gaps for Communicating Risk in Public Health Emergencies [1].

Comics could also be an important way to teach patients important skills such as asking for clarification. When presented with short and easy language accompanied by simple visuals, patients may more readily understand information [2]. In the instance of a complex virus, such as SARS-CoV-2, a simple diagram of the infected area or the virus itself may prove useful. Instead of relying upon verbal communication exclusively, simple visuals may facilitate understanding leading to higher treatment adherence, improved patient satisfaction, and a nurturing clinician-patient relationship [3]. The use of visuals, such as comics, could also be a way to mitigate fear and help patients remember vital information. Along with aiding in the mitigation of fear, humor can also aid in recall [4]. Comics for example, may be more readily able to use funny phrases and mnemonics to explain conditions.

Health communication is not a new area of research; however, there is always need for improvement as doctor-patient communication may be correlated to patient health [5]. While not always the focal point of healthcare, health communication has been recognized as needing continuous study [6]. Medical communication is considered so important that the Accreditation Council for Graduate Medical Education has made it a priority, explaining that practitioners should be able to have the ability to effectively communicate with patients as well as their care teams [7].

Motivation for this study comes from the need to improve health communication through the exploration of under-utilized modalities, such as comics, as called for by the WHO. It is hypothesized that comics could be a workable modality for health communication, in general, as well as during public health crises. As effective communication may encourage the clinician-patient relationship, improve treatment adherence, and raise patient satisfaction—communication, including that of comics, may be considered a ubiquitous tool for pandemic containment.

2. Communication and bioethics

To provide context for the following methodology and how it relates to visual analysis, biomedical ethics, and health communication, attention will be given to the theories and principles from which they come. These theories provide the scope that is used to assess if comics could fulfill, in part or in whole, the WHO's call for continued study of health information in public health crises. One such theory is that of biomedical ethics. Ethical practice is of utmost importance in medicine—and not just in a scientific context, but in areas such as health communication. The four bioethical principles as defined by T. Beauchamp and J. Childress [8] state that physicians have specific duties to their patients. Everything that a physician does must show beneficence; it must be done in an effort to benefit the patient. All actions physicians and clinicians take must be non-maleficent; they must not allow harm to come upon the patient under their watch. Patients need to feel autonomous; that is, doctors need to allow patients' input and narrative in their healthcare processes. Practitioners must always act justly; patients of all kinds have the right to be treated equally.

While these ethical principles have been the standard in healthcare for many years, their scope is more often applied to medical procedures and clinical visits. It has been argued that all aspects of health, including communication, fall under the scope of bioethical principles [9]. Upon the bioethical groundwork laid by ethicists Beauchamp and Childress [10], continuous research is important. One outlet of continuous research is the application of biomedical ethical principles to health communication.

While health communication has been extensively studied, the direct combination of biomedical ethics and communicative maxims has yet to be exhaustively explored. One governing philosophy within the study of communication are the communicative maxims as defined by philosopher H.P. Grice, which serve as dicta for effective communication [11]. Similar to bioethical principles, these four maxims describe what a communicator is obligated to do. Communicators must be mindful of quantity; that is, communicators should not give too much or too little information. The quality of the communication is important as well; it must be truthful. Along with truthfulness, effective communication needs to be relevant; communication should focus on the task at hand. Manner is also of huge importance in communication; the context in which one communicates must be reflected in manner. These four communicative maxims, when combined with the biomedical ethical principles, serve as a foundation for this analysis of health communication. Just as communication must be appropriate in manner, relevance, quantity, and quality, it must also uphold the bioethical principles of beneficence, non-maleficence, autonomy, and justice.

While extending the scope of bioethics to include health communication, it is important to note that communication comes in many forms including comics. The study of communicative value in visuals, such as comics, may be performed using a semiotic lens. This study will assess the effectiveness of a collection of COVID-19 comics as potential tools for health communication. There are three layers to visual communication [12]: the representational, which focuses on the people, places, and objects; the interpersonal, which focuses on the creator, viewers, and characters within the image; and the compositional, which looks at the effectiveness of the composition of an image as a whole [13]. Within the semiotics of comics, there are several modalities of communication, including but not limited to facial expressions, vectors, physical proximity, and ellipses. Each of these visual facets provides meaning to a comic.

Facial expressions can bear important information; there are certain facial expressions that are iconic and may be interpreted across cultural boundaries [14], including sadness, happiness, and anger. These expressions can be used in comics to make meaning and invite understanding. Furthermore, colors play a significant role in the interpretation of images [15, 16], as colors may be associated with different emotions or ideas across cultures. Characters within visuals may also reveal information through vectors and physical proximity [17]. Vectors are lines created through gazes and gestures that serve to direct the viewer's attention to a specific part of an image. The distance of a character's placement within a visual also tells a story: the physical proximity of a person or an object within an image allows the viewer to interpret different relations [18]. For example, a person portrayed with close proximity within an image may be inviting the viewer to create a closer bond with this character. Ellipses are another way to create meaning within an image. Ellipses are intentional blank spaces within visuals that may allow the viewer of an image to use their own imagination to fill that space [19]; allowing the user to fill the space inevitably creates a closer image-viewer connection through interaction.

All of these semiotic modalities within comics have a micro-cognitive effect. Regardless as to whether or not patients are aware of these modalities, they could help lead to positive outcomes. The SARS-CoV-2 pandemic has demonstrated that the control of health communication is just as vital as the containment of the virus itself. While addressing the need for a multimodal approach to health communication, this semiotic analysis studies the effectiveness of comics as a means of such as an approach.

3. Analysis of communicative value and bioethical observance

Now that semiotics, biomedical ethics, and communicative maxims have been reviewed, this research combines these theories to form a theoretical lens for analysis. This theoretical lens analyzes communicative value or communication elements that aid in understanding, within this collection of COVID-19 editorial cartoons. These elements of communicative value will then be further assessed to determine if they can be successfully used within health communication in accordance with communicative maxims and bioethical principles. This research was inspired by the need to continuously study health communication in general as determined by the ACGME, and more specifically to explore new modalities that aid effectual communication during global health crises and pandemics, as called for by the WHO.

In the exploration of new modalities of communication during public health crises, this analysis examines a previously untouched data set, *comics depicting the SARS-CoV-2 pandemic,* in an attempt to describe any potential communicative value that may be adapted for health communication in the future. This collection of *Q&A* style comics are part of an internationally syndicated comic series titled *Health Capsules.* Currently drawn by Bron Smith, these cartoons were originally conceived by Dr. Michael Petti and illustrated by Jud Hurd. These cartoons can be found on the publisher's website [20]. In general, *Health Capsules* answers everyday questions about health and wellness topics, such as exercise, when to visit a physician, allied health practices, symptoms and illnesses, and cultural notions surrounding one's health.

This collection of *Health Capsules* contains four comics that illustrate the COVID-19 pandemic, its causes, and its symptoms. This analysis is founded on the principle that health communication must adhere to bioethical standards under the scope of communicative maxims to be considered effective [21]. With the hypothesis that visual modalities may be an effective means to adhering to such standards, each semiotic element contained within the visuals will be dissected to understand further such element's implicit meaning as may be interpreted by the viewer.

The analysis will begin using a semiotic framework to examine all meaning-making modalities within the comics before proceeding to a bioethical and communicative analysis. Semiotic analysis of these COVID-19 comics will follow a visual analytic framework (**Table 2**) that questions the visual representations within, the emotional connections of, and the overall effectiveness of the visual. After this semiotic analysis to assess for communicative value, a biomedical and communicative analysis will be applied. This analysis will question whether or not the comics are appropriate in manner, relevance, quality, and quantity, and if they adhere to the beneficence of the patient, non-maleficence within medicine, a respect for autonomy, and the upholding of justice. This second step of the analysis is formed on the philosophies of the biomedical ethical principles and the communicative maxims described by H.P. Grice, T. Beauchamp, and J. Childress, and is summarized in a rubric created by J. de Rothewelle in 2019 (**Table 3**).

Visual Representations	Who are the characters present? What medical condition is being represented? Which visual modalities are used to give the comic meaning?
Emotional Connections	What emotional connections are created with the reader? What room is provided for the patient to imagine or create their own narrative? Which visual modalities are used to help emotional connections?
Overall Effectiveness	Overall, how effective is the comic as a tool for medical communication? How does the comic use language to facilitate understanding? What tools does it use to aid understanding and memory?

Table 2.
Rubric for Visual Analysis [22].

Does the discourse follow the Four Communicative Maxims?	Does the discourse comply with the Four Bioethical Principles?
1. Manner: Is this communication in a manner that is appropriate within a healthcare setting?	1. Beneficence: Does this communication work toward benefitting the patient?
2. Relevance: Is this form of communication relevant to the task at hand?	2. Non-maleficence: Does this communication disallow harm to the patient?
3. Quality: Is this communication of quality, that is does it provide true information?	3. Respect for Autonomy: Does this communication promote the patient's informed involvement in their health?
4. Quantity: Is this communication appropriate in amount for which the medium requires?	4. Justice: Does this communication represent fair distribution of health services in the community?
*If the answer to any of the above is "*no,*" how might the discourse be altered so as to better fit communicative and ethical standards within health communication?	

Table 3.
Analysis of Communicative Value & Bioethical Observance [23].

4. Summary of findings

Using a semiotic lens to study the ethics and effectiveness of this collection of comics, this analysis has found that they employ various meaning-making modalities that are noteworthy, but would not be effective as health communication in their present form. Noteworthy communicative values as seen in these comics include: vectors, physical proximity, simple language, simple images, humor, and step-by-step instructions. Such semiotic facets within this collection of comics may be used to place emphasis, further explain, and more fully instruct the general public on health issues during a global health crisis. The findings point to the efficacy of comics as a multimodal means of health communication during global health crises as defined by the WHO.

5. Semiotic analysis of health communication: editorial cartoons

5.1 How is coronavirus spread?

In terms of visual elements, this collection of comics contains noteworthy characteristics, but is not thoroughly prepared to be used in a clinical setting. For example, in **Figure 1** there is a character that may be interpreted to be a patient, and if adapted for health communication, this character may be more specifically drawn as a patient. In comics used as health communication, the portrayal of patients, doctors, and other health professionals may allow the viewer to connect more deeply with the information presented [24–27]. Along with developing the use of characters, however, these comics could do more with representing inanimate objects such as medical supplies, procedures, body parts, and illnesses. **Figure 1** represents disease, or its symptoms quite simply: coughing.

Vectors are an important communicative value within comics. Vectors are anything that forms a line of sight directing a motion or movement within an image [28, 29]. In **Figure 1**, an arrow is used to link the name "coronavirus" with its image. In addition, the particles create a vector spraying outward from the patient's nose and mouth. Vectors may help the viewer find the important parts of the image or determine movement within the image. In the first image, the main character sneezes and shoots COVID-19 aerosols in front of him; these particles

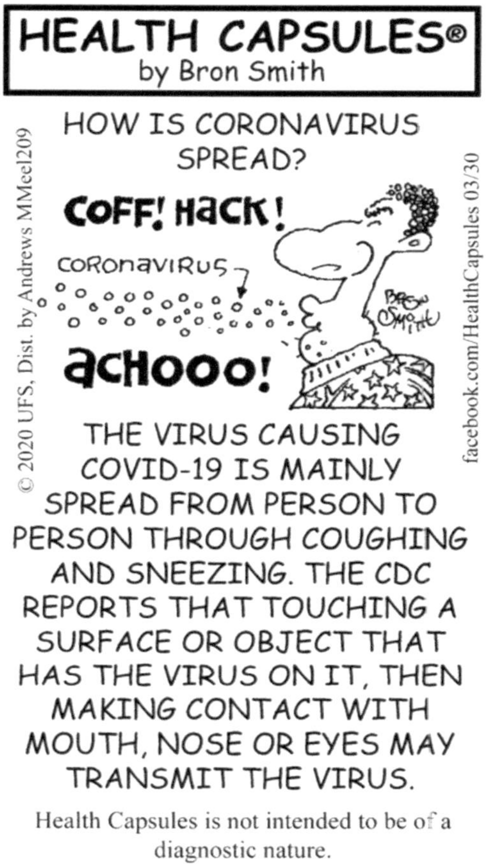
HEALTH CAPSULES®
by Bron Smith
HOW IS CORONAVIRUS SPREAD?
COFF! HACK!
CORONAVIRUS
ACHOOO!
THE VIRUS CAUSING COVID-19 IS MAINLY SPREAD FROM PERSON TO PERSON THROUGH COUGHING AND SNEEZING. THE CDC REPORTS THAT TOUCHING A SURFACE OR OBJECT THAT HAS THE VIRUS ON IT, THEN MAKING CONTACT WITH MOUTH, NOSE OR EYES MAY TRANSMIT THE VIRUS.
Health Capsules is not intended to be of a diagnostic nature.
© 2020 UFS, Dist. by Andrews MMeel209
facebook.com/HealthCapsules 03/30

Figure 1.
How is coronavirus spread?

disseminating from this person are shown to the reader through the use of vectors. Without the use of vectors in this image, one may not understand that COVID-19 aerosols spread via air through the act of coughing.

These comics could be better adapted to suit medical communication by incorporating color. These comics are all black and white, including **Figure 1**; color can convey different moods and emotions [30, 31]; different colors represent universal thoughts or feelings [32]. For example, in many cultures the color white is associated with purity [33], while red is associated with boldness, hastiness, anger, or fear [34, 35]. These colors can be used when incorporated into medical comics by engaging the patient and assisting in the management of feelings and expectations through the use of culturally learned associations with specific colors [36]. For example, in **Figure 1**, color could be used to enhance our understanding of how the character feels: probably feverish which could be portrayed with red or orange-tint colors.

In terms of effectiveness, **Figure 1** is indeed one of the more effective comics in this collection. It explains an illness in concise and non-jargonous language accompanied by a simple image to illustrate the topic. It is easy to understand and may be informational to the patient. For such reasons, lessons of communicative value from this comic may be referenced for future development.

These visuals, along with the use of simple language to explain medical conditions or diagnoses, may be easier for the patient to digest [37, 38]. Furthermore, the link between visuals and memory is well established and thus may aid in recall of this material in the future [39–41]. This is illustrated in **Figure 1**, as the character in the comic is portrayed as coughing, and COVID-19 aerosol particles are shown moving in a projectile motion in front of the character. By using simple visuals instead of complex language in trying to explain COVID-19's ability to spread when someone coughs, it is easier for the patient to understand through the simple image of projectile particles.

Overall, in **Figure 1**, the manner in which information is disseminated is appropriate for the medium used. With a comic as the medium of transmission, simple language is indeed appropriate. This comic presents quality information, which enables patients to make informed decisions. Information of quality allows the patient to retain their autonomy— the information is easy to understand, therefore aiding the patient in making informed decisions.

When examining the quantity of health information distributed among patients within their communities, it is important to consider the biomedical ethical principle of justice [42]. It can be determined whether or not the spread of such information upholds this principle, depending on whether the information shared with one group of patients is drastically different than what is shared with another group of patients. That is not to say that information should not be specifically created and modified for individual groups of patients to best suit their needs; rather, the bioethical principle of justice states that patients across all communities and socioeconomic strata should be treated the same [43]. All patients must receive the same quality of information in a way that is accessible to them, so they can come to appropriate decisions about their health without the privilege of one group over another. Assuming comics developed for use in clinics, hospitals, or outpatient centers alike are not only dispersed in one demographic at the disregard of another, this may be easily avoided.

The relevance of information presented to patients in medicine is highly important: this comic may therefore need an update. Although this collection was not used in a medical context, analysis shows that if it were to be used, the relevance of information would require an update. In particular, **Figure 1** places emphasis on the spread of COVID-19 via surfaces. The CDC has stated that although this is indeed a risk, it is not a central modality of transmission; and so this comic's information may need to be altered to de-emphasize this risk.

5.2 What supplements do doctors recommend for people with COVID-19?

In terms of visual representations, this comic does not detail any specific disease, or symptom. Rather, it is the general asking of questions, as in all *Health Capsules* that may have its own outlet in medicine. Similar to a *Frequently Asked Questions* brochure, comics could be developed to present *FAQ* information to patients more efficiently, understandably, and memorably. In any event, a more effective use would have specifically represented the discourse of the comic in the illustration. Instead of visuals that illustrate the various supplemental treatments, the viewer is presented with an image of a physician.

This image's portrayal of a doctor, who is presumably someone by the name of Dr. Pescatore, a pop-science author and internist, is exclaiming that the size of his nose is too big. Not only is this image seemingly unrelated to the topic being discussed, it may cause confusion to patients who may be led to link COVID-19 symptoms or the taking of supplements to having a big nose. As Dr. Pescatore is not a household name, one would have to research the name to establish the relevance, search if he has written anything about the nose or nasal functions, and then in the final efforts of searching, find images of him to see that he has a large nose; after that process they may still justifiably wonder what this information has to do with anything. Unfortunately, the images and dialogue included with the written text are not on topic for the question that is asked. If comics are to be used in medical care, the images that are accompanying the text should stay on topic and only illustrate what is relevant so as not to confuse patients.

Emotional connections are highly important in healthcare as humans are emotional beings [44]. Therefore, any materials developed to be used in medicine should be aware of the emotional aspect of humanness. In this collection, **Figure 2**'s use of emotion may be helpful to a patient reading it. In **Figure 2**, the character represented is shown clearly smiling, as demonstrated by the curvature of his mouth and the orientation of his eyes. This demonstrates the universal emotion of happiness through facial features. The display of universal emotions through facial features can also help patients feel heard or represented during their care and can serve as an outlet for coping [45].

Not all emotional connections are displayed through facial features. In **Figure 2**, the use of an ominous black space, or ellipsis, to the left of the image is a tool that can help represent fear, discomfort, or the unknown [46]. When seeking medical treatment, patients may be afraid of the unknown [47]. Using an intentionally black space creates a sort of canvas for patients to imagine or even physically draw how they might be feeling or express their worry. In comics that are specifically designed

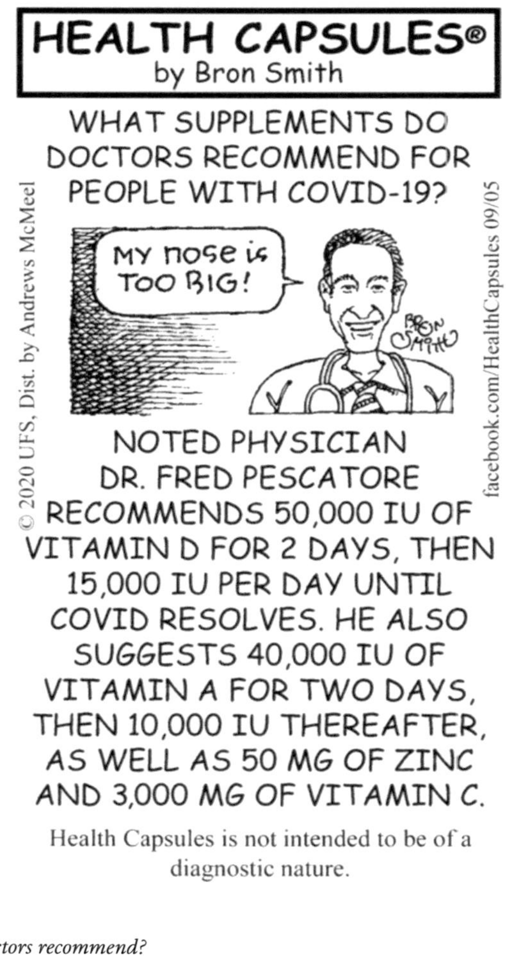
HEALTH CAPSULES®
by Bron Smith
WHAT SUPPLEMENTS DO DOCTORS RECOMMEND FOR PEOPLE WITH COVID-19?
MY nose is TOO BIG!
BRON SMITH
NOTED PHYSICIAN DR. FRED PESCATORE RECOMMENDS 50,000 IU OF VITAMIN D FOR 2 DAYS, THEN 15,000 IU PER DAY UNTIL COVID RESOLVES. HE ALSO SUGGESTS 40,000 IU OF VITAMIN A FOR TWO DAYS, THEN 10,000 IU THEREAFTER, AS WELL AS 50 MG OF ZINC AND 3,000 MG OF VITAMIN C.
© 2020 UFS, Dist. by Andrews McMeel
facebook.com/HealthCapsules 09/05
Health Capsules is not intended to be of a diagnostic nature.

Figure 2.
What supplements do doctors recommend?

to be used in medicine, it may be helpful to include areas within the image that are black, blank, or negative space to represent the unknown and allow the patients to realize their own emotions or fears.

Along with helping to mitigate patient fear, humor is another way to aid memory. Comics tend to include humor or catchy slogans and sayings which are more likely to be remembered by the patient. Studies show that information that stands out, as well as information that elicits a response from the receiver, will be more likely remembered [4].

In this collection, the language is relatively simple and concise, and hence, appropriate in manner. However, **Figure 2** represents an exception. In this comic, the language used could be very confusing to a patient who is not familiar with dosages of supplements. To make this language more appropriate in manner, plainer phrases should be used [48, 49]. For example, a simpler phrase, such as "two doses of vitamin C for the duration of the symptoms." Providing such dense information, such as "50,000 IU of vitamin D for two days, then 15,000 IU per day until COVID resolves" could be experienced as unnecessarily confusing, and beyond the scope of a *FAQ-style* comic.

Along with manner is the biomedical ethical principle of beneficence. Following this principle ensures that everything done within a clinical setting aims at benefiting the patient. Therefore, the manner in which medical communication is created and disseminated must also be created with the benefit of the patient in mind. Generally, the manner of information presented in this collection of comics is beneficent toward the patient. The simple level of language and information presented aids the patient by not using language that is too complex to understand. However, in **Figure 2**, it is uncertain as to whether or not the language used would be widely accessible or beneficial.

Altogether, the quality of this information for comics that are not intended to be used in medicine, could be easily adapted. For example, in **Figure 2**, there is information that is unnecessarily confusing. In a clinical environment, it is of importance to have quality information in an accessible modality available for patients. The quantity of information present in **Figure 2** is appropriate; any more information added to this small comic could cause confusion. Relevance and non-maleficence do come in to question in **Figure 2**, however. In **Figure 2**, it is asked which supplements are recommended for people who have COVID-19. The author then proceeds to accompany this text with an image of a doctor stating that his nose is too big: whatever this information is to mean, it is not entirely relevant, or not at all relevant, to the topic attempting to be communicated to patients. The information presented in the visual is vastly different than the topic and text of the comic. From a more extreme standpoint, the inclusion of non-relevant information could be viewed as maleficent.

5.3 Where did the coronavirus originate?

In **Figure 3**, the character pictured is shown in a frustrated or worried state. The portrayal of emotion in health communication may allow the patient to see such emotion and guide them toward coming to terms with their own [50, 51]. Early on in the SARS-CoV-2 pandemic, there was an arousal of worry about wearing face coverings to help prevent the spread of the virus— this character presented with a concerned expression, and asking about the efficacy of his mask, may be highly relatable to those of the general public.

In addition, in **Figure 3** language is written at a level that is accessible to people of lower literacy. However, just as in **Figure 2**, the image and its dialogue are not directly related to the main text of this comic. This could be viewed as highly confusing. Admittedly, the information about face coverings could be viewed as

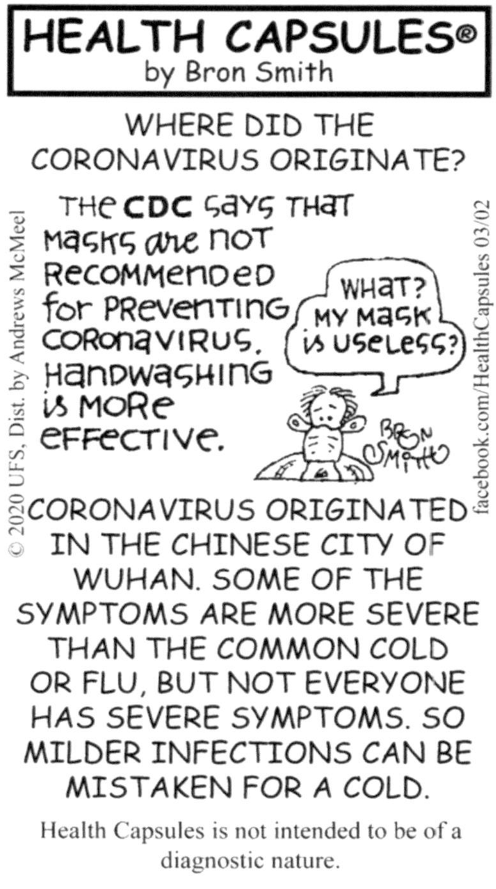
HEALTH CAPSULES®
by Bron Smith
WHERE DID THE CORONAVIRUS ORIGINATE?
THE CDC SAYS THAT MASKS ARE NOT RECOMMENDED FOR PREVENTING CORONAVIRUS. HANDWASHING IS MORE EFFECTIVE.
WHAT? MY MASK IS USELESS?
BRON SMITH
© 2020 UFS, Dist. by Andrews McMeel
facebook.com/HealthCapsules 03/02
CORONAVIRUS ORIGINATED IN THE CHINESE CITY OF WUHAN. SOME OF THE SYMPTOMS ARE MORE SEVERE THAN THE COMMON COLD OR FLU, BUT NOT EVERYONE HAS SEVERE SYMPTOMS. SO MILDER INFECTIONS CAN BE MISTAKEN FOR A COLD.
Health Capsules is not intended to be of a diagnostic nature.

Figure 3.
Where did the coronavirus originate?

important; although, it should warrant a separate panel, so as not to distract from the main text of this comic on the topic of the origin of the coronavirus.

Physical distance between characters within the comic, or between characters and the reader, is another way that comics can create meaning [22, 52]. Depending on how close the characters within the comic are drawn to the outward face of the frame, different social connections can be established. For example, the character in **Figure 3** is drawn from the chest up. Close physical proximity to the reader invites a closer social connection to the characters within the comics. On the other hand, if a medical comic only showed characters far back in the frame with their full bodies in view, from feet to head, distance between the reader and the characters may be interpreted [37, 53]. This may have special implications during the COVID-19 pandemic when citizens are encouraged to *social distance.* The portrayal of characters physically distant from each other could serve to model appropriate behavior.

In terms of quality, there are some inaccuracies within this figure that would need to be properly corrected in order to be used in a medical setting as defined by the communicative maxims [54]. For example, in **Figure 3**, it is stated, "the CDC says masks are not recommended for preventing coronavirus." This comic was created early on in the SARS CoV-2 pandemic when this may have been accurate; however the CDC has since reversed its stance on the subject. At the time of production this *Health Capsule* was appropriate in quality, and therefore lent itself to patient autonomy, though it no longer does so. In addition, this comic is still freely accessible on the internet providing inaccurate information to the non-discerning viewer.

When creating health communication, it is also important to include the proper quantity of information, so as not to confuse the patient. This figure provides only brief information in response to a simple question asked. For this reason, it could be considered appropriate in the quantity of information that it provides. It is important to not give the patient too much information and leave them to sort through what is important or not. Healthcare practitioners must claim that duty and only pass along the information that is important and helpful. Though the quantity of information provided in this figure may be appropriate, other areas like manner and relevancy may need oversight.

In **Figure 3**, in which the origin of the coronavirus is in question, an answer is provided along with an illustration that is off-topic stating that masks are not recommended to be worn during the coronavirus pandemic. While this information could be valuable, it is not relevant to the task at hand within this comic and therefore should be excluded.

Rather, in cases where irrelevant information is presented to patients, it may break the principle of non-maleficence, and harm may come to the patient. In this comic the author states that masks are not recommended for preventing the coronavirus. As this information is no longer relevant to current health guidelines, the spread of this information could have negative effects on the health of the patient. To be non-maleficent and appropriate in relevance, health communication should be updated constantly or removed from circulation.

5.4 Does how I breath affect my risk of Getting COVID?

One valuable semiotic facet from this collection of COVID-19 comics comes from **Figure 4**. This comic gives a brief demonstration of how to breathe more appropriately during the COVID-19 pandemic. Such demonstrations like this may be used to inform a patient how to take their medication correctly or how a surgery will be performed; both of which provide clarity that may ease a patient's fear and aid successful treatment [55–57].

Along with **Figures 1** and **4** is another demonstration of effectiveness in this collection. It explains a health-related topic in plain language and uses visuals to guide the reader toward understanding. Of particular note is the instructional value of providing a step-by-step tutorial for the patient. In this comic, the character is asking the best way to breathe to avoid getting COVID-19. It is unknown if a particular breathing pattern significantly protects someone from contracting the virus. However, this image uses vectors in the form of arrows to demonstrate a movement in medical terms, illustrating breathing in through the nose and out through the mouth. This type of instruction may be highly effective in medical contexts to illustrate and provide clarity on important issues [58–60]. For example, using arrows or vectors can help demonstrate how a diabetic patient experiencing lower extremity swelling should keep their feet elevated until the swelling goes down.

Of course, quality health communication must be evidence based. In this *Health Capsule*, it is asked how breathing effects the risk of contracting COVID-19. After brief research, no readily-available clinical evidence on the effects of how one's breathing affects their contraction of COVID-19 has been found. Information and any materials distributed to patients must be checked for accuracy, clarity, and comprehensiveness, which requires the use of clinically proven information only.

The quality of information presented in medical settings is important when respecting the autonomy of the patient [61]. If the patient is not presented with correct information, it disregards their ability to be actively and informatively involved

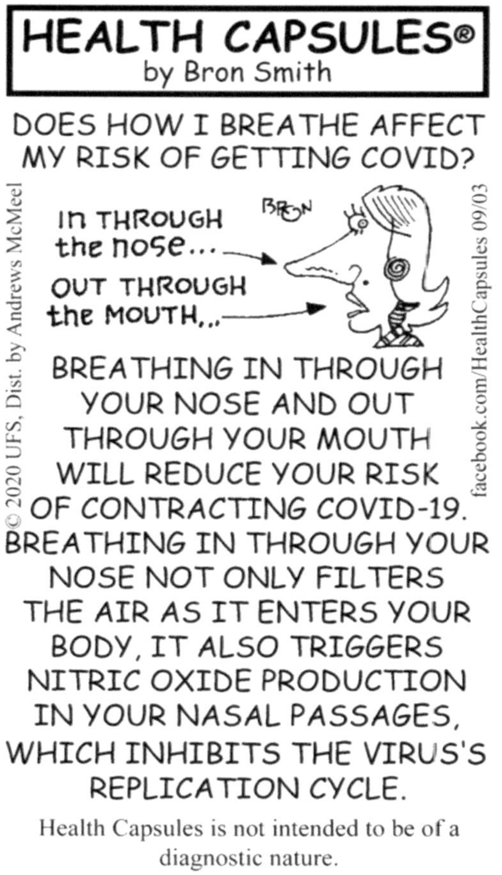

Figure 4.
Does how I breath affect my risk?

in their medical experience. As previously discussed, the quality of information presented within this collection of comics could be quite confusing and, in some places, is outdated or clinically unverifiable. If this collection were to be used in its current form in a clinical setting, the patient would not be able to achieve perfect autonomy in their health.

In health communication, relevance is of key importance, as information that is not relevant could allow harm to the patient [62]. This communicative maxim is aligned with the biomedical principle of non-maleficence. By presenting information that is relevant to the patient, and in support of the task at hand, it helps ensure the patient's safety. **Figure 4**, may present information that could cause harm. Should this information be taken too literally, a patient may believe that simply by breathing in through their nose they can avoid contracting COVID-19, which is of course a misconstrual of information.

6. Discussion

Through the analysis of this collection of *Health Capsules* on COVID-19 as a whole, several characteristics that would be beneficial to health communication were identified. The analysis of these comics reveals that this form of communication may be effective for transmission of medical information with implications for future use, due to the ability to increase patient understanding and recall [63–65]. These images are highly accessible to the average patient and are emotionally relatable [66]. As a response to the WHO's request for health communication research during a pandemic, this analysis posits that comics could be used as successful means of communication during public health crises because of their simplicity.

In the context of health communication, it should be readily apparent that medical comics must uphold communicative principles to be most effective in their effort to provide information to patients. Furthermore, properly vetted communication is of even more importance in medicine; if incorrect or irrelevant information is provided, bodily harm may behold the patient. For this reason, communication's potential to directly inflict harm on patients, health communication must meet biomedical ethical standards. The biomedical ethical principles state that no harm should be inflicted upon the patient. To include medical comics under the scope of health communication, it is evident that medical comics must encourage communicative and medical ethics.

Furthermore, as comics create meaningful discourse through the use of semiotics, such visual semiotic elements need to be payed appropriate attention. Semiotics show that meaning may be gathered from any part of a visual; therefore it is important that patients gather the correct meaning from what they read. Just as verbal language has its own syntactical practices, it may be beneficial for medical comics to have the same level of standardization. With the application of biomedical ethics to health communication, and comics specifically, standards must be set in order to prevent unnecessary confusion or harm. The syntax of comics has already been developed in the field of comics scholarship, as evidenced in this chapter; however, the structure and function comics as a form of health communication could benefit from further study and recommendations of best practices for their use.

As semiotic elements can create emotional connections through facial expressions, invite patient participation through ellipses, set tone through physical proximities, direct the reader's eye though vectors, aid patient recall through humor, increase comprehension through simple language, and guide patients through step-by-step instruction, they are valuable modalities within health communication, so long as they are submitted to bioethical oversight.

6.1 Emotional connections

Creating emotional connections through facial expressions may aid in connecting with the patient, as some expressions are easily recognizable and relatable [67]. For example, a patient may be portrayed as displaying anger; since this emotion transcends culture and may be treated as an iconic facial display, a patient may see this image and be able to make a stronger connection with the comic and the information contained within it. Other iconic facial expressions, such as happiness and sadness, may also be incorporated into health communication to facilitate patient understanding [68]. Relatable information may be very useful in health communication. Due to comics high accessibility, they may be a perfect modality to accomplish this. The representation of patients in medical comics may help patients feel more understood. For example, the use of angry, sad, or happy facial expressions, viewed within this collection, in a medical comic on coping with a terminal cancer diagnosis could help the patient feel justified in their emotions through the stages of their illness. The simple feeling of being understood and emotionally supported could improve the medical experience [69].

6.2 Patient participation

Patient participation may be invited through an ellipsis, or an intentional black or blank space within the image that the patient is free to fill in [70]. As interpreted from this discussion, this may allow the patient to take an active role in medical literature that may be overly focused on diagnosing or prescribing. Allowing patients to take an active role in their illness narrative has shown to increase healing and patient satisfaction [71]. In medicine, diagnosing a patient often inadvertently prescribes the patient an illness narrative; allowing the patient to be the creator of their own illness narrative and empowering them to visualize it for themselves may be an important technique to help patients find their role or their voice in their treatment [72]. For example, in a comic about a diagnosis of major depression, a panel could be left blank with a prompt encouraging the patient to draw or write how they feel. Or, in this same situation, a comic panel could be completely blackened, with a prompt asking the patient to close their eyes and imagine what this diagnosis looks like to them. These modalities allow the patient to take a more active role in their illness narrative and could also serve as a therapeutic outlet of expression.

6.3 Physical proximity

Setting tone through physical proximities could be another way to create meaning within comics as a form of health communication. This collection of comics portrayed all characters in close physical proximity– from the chest up— which may serve to create a stronger bond between characters and readers [73]. Medical practice and hospitals could be viewed as a cold experience [74, 75]; throughout such bodily positioning, the reader of medical comics is invited to make a stronger connection with what they are reading [76]. It is arguably a small difference compared to the interpersonal relationship between the patient and the doctor, but if the patient could feel more welcomed or more understood through the positioning of characters represented through visual medical literature, it may be viewed as enhancing the overall medical experience. In addition to creating a closer connection with the patient, the strategic placement of characters in comics may also portray important values. In this analysis, for example, characters placed front and center in visuals were observed. In situations where the patient may often feel overlooked, by placing the patient front and center in a visual— when the patient may not feel centrally important in their own illness experience— the patient may feel acknowledged as the center of their care.

6.4 Vectors

Directing the reader's eye though vectors guides the line of sight in certain directions to place emphasis [77]. This visual technique to portray meaning could be successfully adapted to place emphasis within comics in health communication. For example, as demonstrated in *Health Capsules*, a patient may be reading a medical comic about obesity, and instead of placing emphasis on the various symptoms depicted, vectors could be illustrated through placement of images to place emphasis on the underlying cause. For example, a comic depicting obesity could demonstrate the symptoms and emotionally acknowledge the frustrations a patient may be experiencing, while at the same time directing the reader's eye toward solutions, such as physical exercise and moderation of food intake. Whether or not a patient is cognizant of the fact that their attention is being directed in this way may not matter; what matters is the microcognitive process that follows in which the patient may subconsciously classify the object to which their attention is being drawn, such as physical activity, as more important.

6.5 Patient recall, mitigation of fear

Aiding patient recall through humor, as a distinct type of emotional connection, may increase the memorization of information presented to patients [78]. As observed in this analysis, the use of humor may make information easier to remember and may help mitigate a patient's fear [79]. Along with information that stands out to the patient, health information that is clear and concise may be easier for patients to remember. For example, in a comic about extreme anxiety about hospital visits, the patient could be encouraged to breathe deeply through some sort of humorous approach, which would then be more likely remembered for future visits.

6.6 Simple language

Increasing comprehension through simple language is one of the easiest adaptations that can be implemented within health communication. Doctors and other medical practitioners speak their own language of highly specialized terms and codes that must be translated into plain language, so that it is accessible to all patients, as effectively demonstrated in this collection. Comics are a great media to do this, as it is typical and expected that a comic use simple and concise language with an accompanying visual. For example, instead of saying "One should exercise 5 out of 7 days a week for 75 minutes with moderate sweating to increase positive effects on body mass index, mobility, and overall health..." simpler language such as "Get outside and exercise, it's good for your health!" could more effectively reach some audiences.

6.7 Step-by-step instruction

Guiding patients through step-by-step instructions may provide a higher level of ease and less fear of the unknown [80]. For example, it need not take more than two pages to illustrate simply the processes of a laparoscopic procedure. Using comics may also be helpful in prescribing instructions for recovery. This may be especially helpful for non-native speakers of the language of treatment, patients struggling with illiteracy, or patients who are visual learners. For example, rather than verbally instructing a patient on the variety of doses and drugs to take at various times of the day with or without food, visuals may help. A visual that shows the medication type, whether pill, injection, or liquid, how to cut or measure it, perhaps a sun or a moon to depict what time of day to take it at, and illustrations of what to take it with like a meal or water, as was done in a particular case of non-English speakers at a teaching hospital in Merced, California [81], might increase patient understanding and adherence to treatment.

6.8 Asking questions

Step-by-step instructions, as illustrated in *Health Capsules*, may also include teaching patients how to ask questions when something remains unknown. Patients may not ask for clarification for a number of reasons, including fear of appearing unintelligent [82] or difficult [83], fear of a generic answer to an emotional question [84], or simply not knowing how to ask. Comics have a unique opportunity to support this problem. These comics that are in a *Q&A* format and ask simple or funny questions may encourage those viewing these comics to ask any questions they may have. For example, through comics depicting patients asking relatively simple questions to their doctor, patients may realize that questions at all levels, no matter how simple, are important enough to be asked, and thus may encourage patient to seek more information about their health and treatment. Seeking information, asking questions, and receiving adequate answers have been linked to higher patient satisfaction in their healthcare [85–87].

7. Implications for further research

Using a lens founded upon philosophies from semiotics, communication, and biomedical ethics, this analysis examined the communicative value and potential use of SARS-CoV-2 *Health Capsules* as a modality of health communication in a pandemic. This study was conducted to answer the WHO's call for health communication research during global health crises and emphasizes the importance of health communication in accordance with the ACGME and other stakeholders, coming to several conclusions.

Comics have the potential to communicate appropriately in manner, relevance, quality, and quantity, as well as to disseminate medical information beneficently, justly, non-maleficently, and in a way that supports patient-autonomy. The findings of this analysis show that medical comics could fulfil in part the WHO's search for multimodal methods of health communication during pandemics.

This analysis also demonstrates that comics could be used effectively and ethically to communicate during pandemics and in health communication generally, using semiotic features, such as using facial expressions to create emotional connections, using physical proximities to set tone, using vectors to direct the reader's eye, using humor to aid recall, using simple language to increase comprehension, and using illustrated step-by-step instructions to guide patients. However, without exhaustive research on the topic, there are no current best practices for the creation of biomedically and communicatively ethical medical comics.

The findings of this analysis call for a broader scope of the use of comics in medicine and suggest standardized guidelines for their use. Guidelines that establish regularized uses of facial expressions, ellipses, vectors, physical proximity, humor, step-by-step instructions and other semiotic values typically found within comics, should be established prior to the general and widespread use of comics as means of health communication.

Author details

Jonathan de Rothewelle
Harry S Truman College, United States

*Address all correspondence to: jcomynderothewelle@gmail.com

References

[1] * Summarized from *Communicating risk in public health emergencies:* A WHO guideline for emergency risk communication (ERC) policy and practice. 2017. ISBN 978-92-4-155020-8

[2] Feng, D., and K. L. O'Halloran. 2012. "Representing Emotive Meaning in Visual Images: A Social Semiotic Approach." Journal of Pragmatics 44 (14, November 01): 2067-2084. doi:10.1016/j.pragma.2012.10.003.

[3] Henry SG, Matthias MS. Patient-clinician communication about pain: A conceptual model and narrative review. Pain Medicine. 2018;19(11):2154-2165. DOI: 10.1093/pm/pny003

[4] Tyng CM, Amin HU, Saad MNM, Malik AS. The Influences of Emotion on Learning and Memory. Front Psychol. 2017;8:1454. Published 2017 Aug 24. DOI: 10.3389/fpsyg.2017.01454

[5] Ong LM, de Haes JC, Hoos AM, Lammes FB. Doctor-patient communication: a review of the literature. Soc Sci Med. 1995 Apr;40(7):903-918. doi: 10.1016/0277-9536(94)00155-m. PMID: 7792630.

[6] Ferreira-Padilla G, Ferrández-Antón T, Baleriola-Júlvez J, Braš M, Đorđević V. Communication skills in medicine: where do we come from and where are we going?. Croat Med J. 2015;56(3):311-314. doi:10.3325/cmj.2015.56.311.

[7] (Accreditation Council for Graduate Medical Education 2015).

[8] Beauchamp T, Childress J. Principles of Biomedical Ethics. 6th ed. Oxford University Press; 2009

[9] de Rothewelle, JC. Biomedical Ethics and Communicative Maxims: Case Studies in Outpatient Health. 2020. Intech Open

[10] Beauchamp T, Childress J. Principles of Biomedical Ethics. 6th ed. Oxford University Press; 2009

[11] Grice HP. Logic and conversation. In: Cole P, Morgan JL, editors. Syntax and Semantics, Speech Acts. Vol. 3. New York: Academic Press; 1975. pp. 41-58

[12] Kress G, Van Leeuwen T. Multimodal Discourse: The Modes and Media of Contemporary Communication. Oxford, UK: Oxford University Press; 2001

[13] Kress G, Van Leeuwen T. Multimodal Discourse: The Modes and Media of Contemporary Communication. Oxford, UK: Oxford University Press; 2001

[14] Forceville, C. Visual Representations of the Idealized Cognitive Model of Anger in the Asterix Album La Zizanie. Journal of Pragmatics 37: 69-88. doi:10.1016/j.pragma.2003.10.002.

[15] K. Yildirim, A. Akalin-Baskaya, M.L. Hidayetoglu, Effects of indoor color on mood and cognitive performance, Building and Environment, Volume 42, Issue 9, 2007, Pages 3233-3240,

[16] Wilms, L., Oberfeld, D. Color and emotion: effects of hue, saturation, and brightness. Psychological Research 82, 896-914 (2018). https://doi.org/10.1007/s00426-017-0880-8

[17] Lister, M., and L. Wells. 2000. Seeing beyond Belief: Cultural Studies as an Approach to Analyzing the Visual. In The Handbook of Visual Analysis, 61-91, eds T. Van Leeuwen and C. Jewitt. London: Sage. 2001.

[18] Kress G, Van Leeuwen T. Multimodal Discourse: The Modes and Media of Contemporary

Communication. Oxford, UK: Oxford University Press; 2001

[19] Harrison, C. 2003. "Visual Social Semiotics: Understanding How Still Images Make Meaning." Technical Communication 50 (1): 46-60.

[20] www.gocomics.com, Copywrite Andrew McMeel Universal 2020.

[21] de Rothewelle, JC. Biomedical Ethics and Communicative Maxims: Case Studies in Outpatient Health. 2020. Intech Open

[22] de Rothewelle, JC. Visual Pathologies: The Semiotics of the Patient and the Practitioner in Comics. 2019 Intech open

[23] de Rothewelle, JC. Biomedical Ethics and Communicative Maxims: Case Studies in Outpatient Health. 2020. Intech Open

[24] Green MJ. Graphic storytelling and medical narrative: The use of comics in medical education. In: The Graphic Medicine Manifesto. University Park, Pennsylvania: The Pennsylvania State University Press; 2015

[25] Czerwiec MK. Taking Turns: Stories from HIV/AIDS Care Unit 371. University Park, Pennsylvania: The Pennsylvania State University Press; 2017

[26] Chute H. Comics as literature? Reading graphic narrative. PMLA [Internet]. 2008 Mar;123(2):452-465. DOI: 10.1632/pmla.2008.123.2.452

[27] Bateman JA. Text and Image. Abingdon, United Kingdom: Routledge; 2014 May. DOI: 10.4324/9781315773971

[28] Kaplan-Weinger J. Addressing loss and resilience: Informing patient care through comic narratives. Atrium: The Report of the Northwestern Medical Humanities and Bioethics Program. Evanston, Illinois: Northwestern Center for Bioethics; 2012;(10)

[29] Juricevic I, Hcity orvath AJ. Analysis of motions in comic book cover art: Using pictorial metaphors. Comics Grid: Journal of Comics Scholarship [Internet]. 2016 Apr;6(1). DOI: 10.16995/cg.71

[30] K. Yildirim, A. Akalin-Baskaya, M.L. Hidayetoglu, Effects of indoor color on mood and cognitive performance, Building and Environment, Volume 42, Issue 9, 2007, Pages 3233-3240,

[31] Wilms, L., Oberfeld, D. Color and emotion: effects of hue, saturation, and brightness. Psychological Research 82, 896-914 (2018). https://doi.org/10.1007/s00426-017-0880-8

[32] Andrew J. Elliot and Markus A. Maier Color Psychology: Effects of Perceiving Color on Psychological Functioning in Humans Annual Review of Psychology 2014 65:1, 95-120

[33] Sherman GD, Clore GL. 2009. White and black are perceptual symbols of moral purity and pollution. Psychol. Sci. 20:1019-25

[34] Hill RA, Barton RA. 2005. Red enhances human performance in contests. Nature 435:293

[35] Pryke SR. 2009. Is red an innate or learned signal of aggression and intimidation? Anim. Behav. 78:393-398

[36] de Rothewelle, JC. Biomedical Ethics and Communicative Maxims: Case Studies in Outpatient Health. 2020. Intech Open

[37] de Rothewelle, JC. Comics and medical narrative: a visual semiotic dissection of graphic medicine. 2018. Journal of Graphic Novels and Comics. Routledge.

[38] Williams ICM. Graphic medicine: comics as medical narrative. Medical Humanities [Internet]. 2012 Jan;38(1):21-27. DOI: 10.1136/medhum-2011-010093

[39] Brewer, W. F.: What is autobiographical memory? In D. Rubin (Ed.), Autobiographical Memory (pp. 25-Cambridge: Cambridge University Press, 1986.

[40] Brewer, W. F.: Qualitative analysis of the recalls of randomly sampled autobiographical events. In M. M. Gruneberg, P. E. Morris, & R. N. Sykes (Eds.), Practical Aspects of Memory: Current Research and Issues (Vol. 1, pp. 263-268). Chichester: Wiley, 1988.

[41] van Weert JC, van Noort G, Bol N, van Dijk L, Tates K, Jansen J. Tailored information for cancer patients on the Internet: effects of visual cues and language complexity on information recall and satisfaction. Patient Educ Couns. 2011 Sep;84(3):368-378. doi: 10.1016/j.pec.2011.04.006. Epub 2011 May 8. PMID: 21550757.

[42] Beauchamp T, Childress J. Principles of Biomedical Ethics. 6th ed. Oxford University Press; 2009

[43] Beauchamp T, Childress J. Principles of Biomedical Ethics. 6th ed. Oxford University Press; 2009

[44] Billington, J. 2016. Is Literature Healthy? Oxford, United Kingdom: Oxford University Press.

[45] jmh.2010.005603. Feng, D., and K. L. O'Halloran. 2012. "Representing Emotive Meaning in Visual Images: A Social Semiotic Approach." Journal of Pragmatics 44 (14, November 01): 2067-2084. doi:10.1016/j. pragma.2012.10.003.

[46] Harrison, C. 2003. "Visual Social Semiotics: Understanding How Still Images Make Meaning." Technical Communication 50 (1): 46-60.

[47] Hills LS. Working with anxious or fearful patients: a training tool for the medical practice staff. J Med Pract Manage. 2007 Jul-Aug;23(1):50-53. PMID: 17824264.

[48] Linder, D., Dall'Olio, E., Gisondi, P. et al. Perception of Disease and Doctor-Patient Relationship Experienced by Patients with Psoriasis. AM J Clin Dermatol 10, 325-330 (2009). https://doi.org/10.2165/11311190-000000000-00000

[49] Shaw A, Ibrahim S, Reid F, Ussher M, Rowlands G. Patients' perspectives of the doctor-patient relationship and information giving across a range of literacy levels. Patient Educ Couns. 2009 Apr;75(1):114-120. doi: 10.1016/j.pec.2008.09.026. Epub 2008 Nov 28. PMID: 19041210.

[50] Kaplan-Weinger J. Addressing loss and resilience: Informing patient care through comic narratives. Atrium: The Report of the Northwestern Medical Humanities and Bioethics Program. Evanston, Illinois: Northwestern Center for Bioethics; 2012;(10)

[51] jmh.2010.005603. Feng, D., and K. L. O'Halloran. 2012. "Representing Emotive Meaning in Visual Images: A Social Semiotic Approach." Journal of Pragmatics 44 (14, November 01): 2067-2084. doi:10.1016/j. pragma.2012.10.003.

[52] Kaplan-Weinger J. Addressing loss and resilience: Informing patient care through comic narratives. Atrium: The Report of the Northwestern Medical Humanities and Bioethics Program. Evanston, Illinois: Northwestern Center for Bioethics; 2012;(10)

[53] Kress, G., and T. Van Leeuwen. 2006. Reading Images: The Grammar of Visual Design. London & New York: Routledge.

[54] Grice HP. Logic and conversation. In: Cole P, Morgan JL, editors. Syntax

and Semantics, Speech Acts. Vol. 3. New York: Academic Press; 1975. pp. 41-58

[55] Mohan A, Riley MB, Boyington D, Kripalani S. PictureRx: Illustrated medication instructions for patients with limited health literacy. J Am Pharm Assoc (2003). 2012;52(5):e122-e129. doi:10.1331/JAPhA.2012.11132

[56] Delp C, Jones J. Communicating information to patients: the use of cartoon illustrations to improve comprehension of instructions. Acad Emerg Med. 1996 Mar;3(3):264-270. doi: 10.1111/j.1553-2712.1996.tb03431.x. PMID: 8673784.

[57] Kripalani S, Robertson R, Love-Ghaffari MH, Henderson LE, Praska J, Strawder A, Katz MG, Jacobson TA. Development of an illustrated medication schedule as a low-literacy patient education tool. Patient Educ Couns. 2007 Jun;66(3):368-377. doi: 10.1016/j.pec.2007.01.020. Epub 2007 Mar 6. PMID: 17344015.

[58] Mohan A, Riley MB, Boyington D, Kripalani S. PictureRx: Illustrated medication instructions for patients with limited health literacy. J Am Pharm Assoc (2003). 2012;52(5):e122-e129. doi:10.1331/JAPhA.2012.11132

[59] Delp C, Jones J. Communicating information to patients: the use of cartoon illustrations to improve comprehension of instructions. Acad Emerg Med. 1996 Mar;3(3):264-270. doi: 10.1111/j.1553-2712.1996.tb03431.x. PMID: 8673784.

[60] Kripalani S, Robertson R, Love-Ghaffari MH, Henderson LE, Praska J, Strawder A, Katz MG, Jacobson TA. Development of an illustrated medication schedule as a low-literacy patient education tool. Patient Educ Couns. 2007 Jun;66(3):368-377. doi: 10.1016/j.pec.2007.01.020. Epub 2007 Mar 6. PMID: 17344015.

[61] Beauchamp T, Childress J. Principles of Biomedical Ethics. 6th ed. Oxford University Press; 2009

[62] Beauchamp T, Childress J. Principles of Biomedical Ethics. 6th ed. Oxford University Press; 2009

[63] Brewer, W. F.: What is autobiographical memory? In D. Rubin (Ed.), Autobiographical Memory (pp. 25-Cambridge: Cambridge University Press, 1986.

[64] Brewer, W. F.: Qualitative analysis of the recalls of randomly sampled autobiographical events. In M. M. Gruneberg, P. E. Morris, & R. N. Sykes (Eds.), Practical Aspects of Memory: Current Research and Issues (Vol. 1, pp. 263-268). Chichester: Wiley, 1988.

[65] van Weert JC, van Noort G, Bol N, van Dijk L, Tates K, Jansen J. Tailored information for cancer patients on the Internet: effects of visual cues and language complexity on information recall and satisfaction. Patient Educ Couns. 2011 Sep;84(3):368-378. doi: 10.1016/j.pec.2011.04.006. Epub 2011 May 8. PMID: 21550757.

[66] Chute H. Comics as literature? Reading graphic narrative. PMLA [Internet]. 2008 Mar;123(2):452-465. DOI: 10.1632/pmla.2008.123.2.452

[67] Forceville, C. Visual Representations of the Idealized Cognitive Model of Anger in the Asterix Album La Zizanie. Journal of Pragmatics 37: 69-88. doi:10.1016/j.pragma.2003.10.002.

[68] Forceville, C. Visual Representations of the Idealized Cognitive Model of Anger in the Asterix Album La Zizanie. Journal of Pragmatics 37: 69-88. doi:10.1016/j.pragma.2003.10.002.

[69] Halpern, J. 2003. "What Is Clinical Empathy? Jgim." Journal of

General Internal Medicine 18:670-674. doi:10.1046/j.1525-1497.2003.21017.x.

[70] Harrison, C. 2003. "Visual Social Semiotics: Understanding How Still Images Make Meaning." Technical Communication 50 (1): 46-60.

[71] Frank, A., . W. 2013. The Wounded Storyteller. Body, Illness & Ethics. Second ed. Chicago; London: University of Chicago Press.

[72] Foucault M. The Birth of the Clinic. Routledge; 2002 Nov. DOI: 10.4324/9780203406373

[73] Kaplan-Weinger J. Addressing loss and resilience: Informing patient care through comic narratives. Atrium: The Report of the Northwestern Medical Humanities and Bioethics Program. Evanston, Illinois: Northwestern Center for Bioethics; 2012;(10)

[74] Kompanje, E.J.O., van Mol, M.M. & Nijkamp, M.D. 'I just have admitted an interesting sepsis'. Do we dehumanize our patients?. Intensive Care Med 41, 2193-2194 (2015). https://doi.org/10.1007/s00134-015-4014-8

[75] Haque, O., & Waytz, A. (2012). Dehumanization in Medicine: Causes, Solutions, and Functions. Perspectives on Psychological Science, 7(2), 176-186. Retrieved November 18, 2020, from http://www.jstor.org/stable/41613554

[76] Kress G, Van Leeuwen T. Reading Images. Routledge; 2006 Mar. DOI: 10.4324/9780203619728

[77] Lister, M., and L. Wells. 2000. Seeing beyond Belief: Cultural Studies as an Approach to Analyzing the Visual. In The Handbook of Visual Analysis, 61-91, eds T. Van Leeuwen and C. Jewitt. London: Sage. 2001.

[78] Tyng CM, Amin HU, Saad MNM, Malik AS. The Influences of Emotion on Learning and Memory. Front Psychol. 2017;8:1454. Published 2017 Aug 24. doi:10.3389/fpsyg.2017.01454

[79] Nezlek, J. B., & Derks, P. (2001). Use of humor as a coping mechanism, psychological adjustment, and social interaction, HUMOR, 14(4), 395-413. doi: https://doi.org/10.1515/humr.2001.011

[80] Hills LS. Working with anxious or fearful patients: a training tool for the medical practice staff. J Med Pract Manage. 2007 Jul-Aug;23(1):50-53. PMID: 17824264.

[81] Fadiman, A. he Spirit Catches You and You Fall Down: A Hmong Child, Her American Doctors, and the Collision of Two Cultures. FSG Classics. 2012

[82] Hills LS. Working with anxious or fearful patients: a training tool for the medical practice staff. J Med Pract Manage. 2007 Jul-Aug;23(1):50-53. PMID: 17824264.

[83] Authoritarian Physicians And Patients' Fear Of Being Labeled 'Difficult' Among Key Obstacles To Shared Decision Making Dominick L. Frosch, Suepattra G. May, Katharine A.S. Rendle, Caroline Tietbohl, and Glyn Elwyn Health Affairs 2012 31:5, 1030-1038

[84] Beach WA, Dozier DM. Fears, Uncertainties, and Hopes: Patient-Initiated Actions and Doctors' Responses During Oncology Interviews. J Health Commun. 2015;20(11):1243-1254. doi: 10.1080/10810730.2015.1018644

[85] Korsch BM, Gozzi EK and Francis V (1968) Gaps in doctor–patient communication: doctor patient interaction and patient satisfaction. 855-870

[86] Kupst M, Dresser K, Schulman JL and Paul MH (1975) Evaluation of

methods to improve communication in the physician–patient relationship. 420-429

[87] Brown R, Butow PN, Boyer MJ, Tattersall MH. Promoting patient participation in the cancer consultation: evaluation of a prompt sheet and coaching in question-asking. Br J Cancer. 1999;80(1-2):242-248. doi:10.1038/sj.bjc.6690346

Chapter 7

Building Community and Fostering Health and Well-Being through a Collaborative School Based Project

Abimbola O. Asojo, Hoa Vo, Suyeon Bae,
Chelsea Hetherington, Sarah Cronin and Judy Myers

Abstract

This article presents lessons learned from collaborative service-learning projects aimed at bridging the gap between theory and practice by providing students design experiences in authentic settings. Interior design students gained disciplinary and civic benefits while problem solving for a preK-5 elementary school calming room, dining room, and teacher sanctuary. The elementary school teachers and staff reported the redesigned calming room supported students' emotional and self-regulation skills. Teachers and staff also reported the dining room and teacher sanctuary supported the school community well-being. The authors' present findings and hope the article can serve as a model for educators interested in community building service-learning projects in school environments.

Keywords: Community, collaborative, service-learning, civic benefits, interior design

1. Introduction

Several researchers have presented how community engagement enhances partnerships between the University and the public while providing positive impacts on learning experiences [1, 2]. This article discusses a partnership between a school community and University in the design of the school calming room, dining room, and teacher sanctuary. Calming rooms have been found to support the well-being of children and youth, particularly in improving their self-regulation skills. Calming rooms are spaces that students can retreat to when they feel particularly agitated or dysregulated [3], and trauma-informed care approaches support the creation of such spaces where students can learn to better self-regulate [4–6]. Such spaces utilize design elements that facilitate calming and relaxation, such as soothing colors, like blue, green, and violet color palettes, and minimal stimulation [3, 7]. Calming rooms, or "sensory rooms", have largely been implemented with children and youth in residential psychiatric settings and juvenile justice facilities. For schools, this is a relatively novel approach, with limited empirical research on its impacts. Anecdotally, teachers have reported that calming rooms in schools have led to improvements in self-regulation [4]. Teachers have also reported that children have a positive view of calming rooms as a quiet, peaceful space to retreat to when something is bothering them [8, 9]. As such, improving self-regulation skills, which are often negatively impacted by chronic stress and trauma [10, 11], is a fundamental goal in supporting children's health and well-being. Dining and cafeteria spaces can be another source of influences on students' mood. A friendly, family-like, and collaborative eating environment boosts comfort and relatedness in children [12]. While elementary students can experience the primary effects of trauma and stress, other school personnel also suffer from secondary effects. Teachers and staff are involved in students' development, and in need of health and well-being support [13, 14]. A teacher sanctuary provides space for teachers and staff to refuel and rejuvenate in the school environment.

2. Elementary school calming room project

The University of Minnesota Extension Children, Youth, and Family Consortium collaborated with Bruce Vento, a local elementary school, to capitalize on the strengths of the school and its community in supporting its students [15]. The project partners worked together to identify the biggest areas of need in this East Saint Paul school, which is under-resourced with a diverse student body, many of whom experience chronic stress and behavioral dysregulation. During the process, the implementation of a calming room to provide a space for students to develop self-regulation skills was derived. The University personnel then connected with the Interior design program to join the project partners in the design process. This led to the integration of the calming room project in a sophomore level interior design course at the University of Minnesota in spring 2015 taught by the first author. Interior design students were able to connect directly with the community through site visits and working with the school staff to learn more about the design problem and existing conditions (**Figure 1**).

2.1 The design

The project goal was to redesign the existing institutional looking calming room in Bruce Vento elementary school to foster students' self-regulation. In several days in a design studio course, 23 interior design students worked in groups of three to design a safe place for children to express emotions, develop effective coping skills, and learn self-regulation skills. On day one, students visited the school to meet with the principal, counselor, and teachers in the existing calming room. On day two, students presented their existing space analysis and building system report then developed their concept and schematic designs (2D floor plan and 3D interior vignette sketches) in studio. On day three, students presented their concept and schematic design to the clients and for their feedback. Days four and five were spent in the studio finalizing the design with the instructor's feedback and desk critiques. On day six, students presented finalized design drawings to the school principal, counselor, representatives from the University of Minnesota Extension Children, Youth and Family Consortium, a local architect, instructors, and their peers.

After the presentations, two groups had their design solutions selected and incorporated in the actual space. The first group proposed a design to allow children experience a personal adventure (**Figure 2**). The second student group proposed the space to be a haven for students and enable them to self-regulate quickly, efficiently (**Figure 3**). The implementation of the final calming room (**Figure 4**) was within a limited budget of $4975. A large bean bag chair and four cubbies filled with

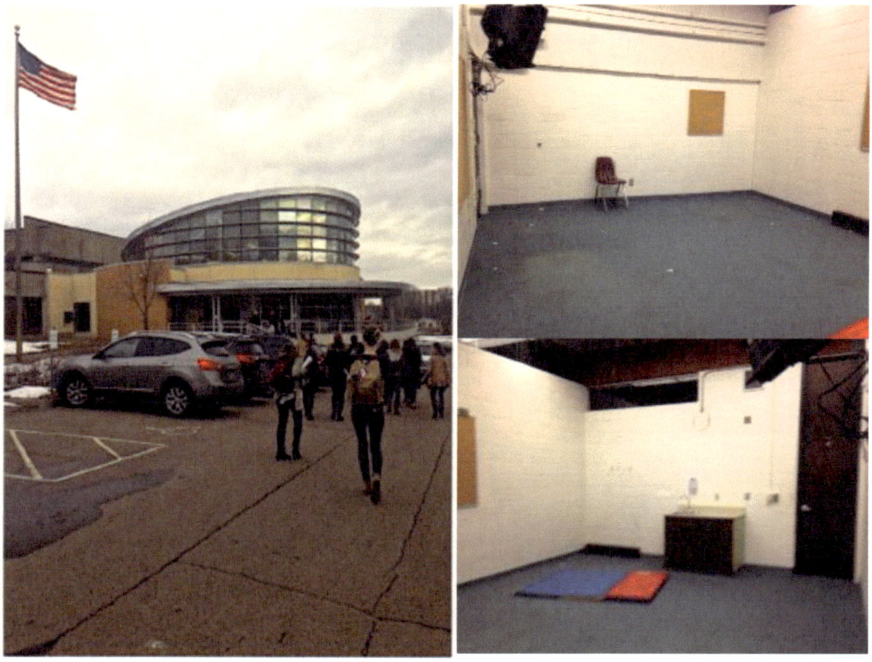

Figure 1.
Bruce Vento School Exterior and former Calming Room Interior Condition (Source: Pictures by Author 1).

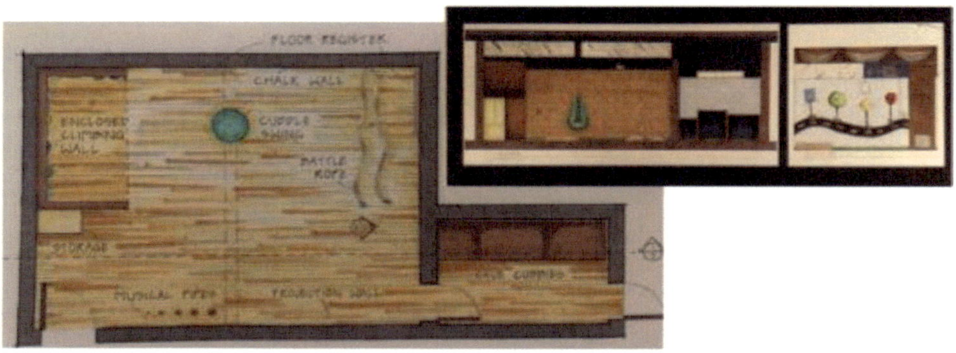

Figure 2.
Design proposal by student team to allow children experience their personal adventure (Source: Emily Devore, James Thoma, and Hailey Wrasman, Spring 2015 IDES 2604 Interior Design IV course).

soft pillows were incorporated in the space to help students relax and regulate their emotions. The cubies provided a crawl and snug space for students. Nature inspired imagery were placed on the wall since the space lacked direct sunlight to provide connection to the natural environment. Cloud ceiling panels were used to soften the harsh fluorescent lighting and the huge rug softened the space and provided connection to nature. The wall labyrinth mural, blues, greens and earth tones colors in the space were used to create a soothing atmosphere for the students. A dark blue color accent on the upper portion of the wall was used to reduce the impact of the high ceiling and make the anthropometric proportion and height of the room more relatable for the students. The simplicity in the new space was to avoid over stimulating the students and help them relax and self-regulate.

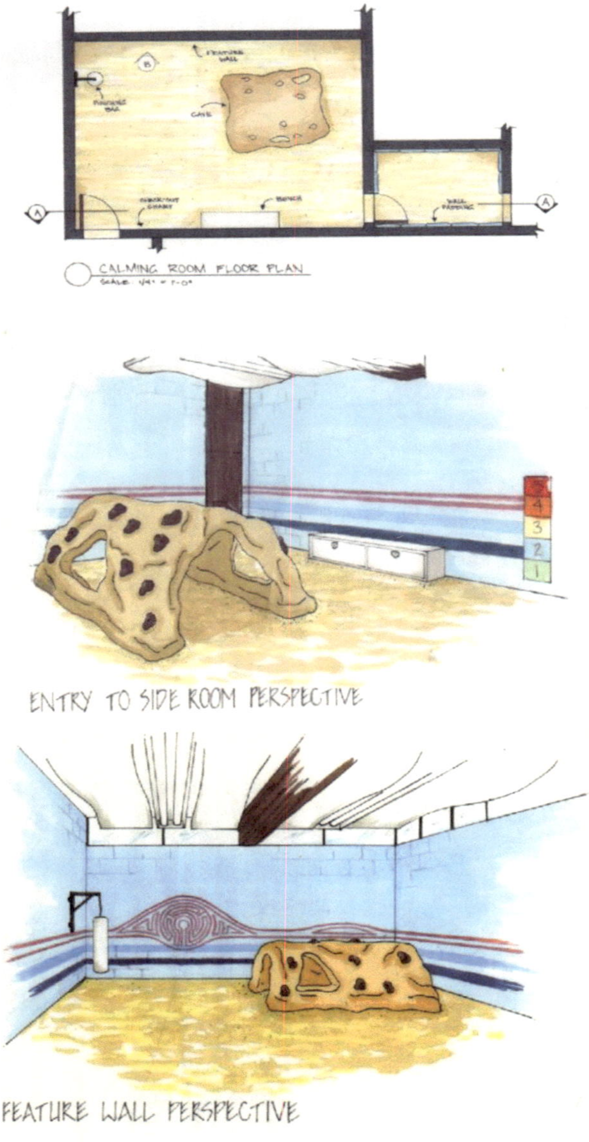

Figure 3.
Design proposal by the student team proposed the space to be a haven for students and enable them to release their anger quickly, efficiently, and safely. Light and dark blues with small amounts of light pink and dull yellow were used to create a tranquil environment. Curved lines were repeated throughout the space to imitate the soft curves of waves and clouds (Source: Rachel Grothe and Hannah Segar, Spring 2015 IDES 2604 Interior Design IV course).

2.2 Evaluation

To study the impact of the redesigned calming room, interviews were conducted with teachers and staff in fall 2016 (n = 20). 11 participants reported being teachers, 5 were behavioral staff (e.g., school social workers), and 4 were other school staff. In the first part of the interview, two interviewers asked teachers and staff to reflect on the impact that the calming room had on students and the school environment. In a second part of the interview, teachers and staff were asked about the impact of other aspects of the partnership, though those results are not detailed here. Interviews were then transcribed and coded for themes.

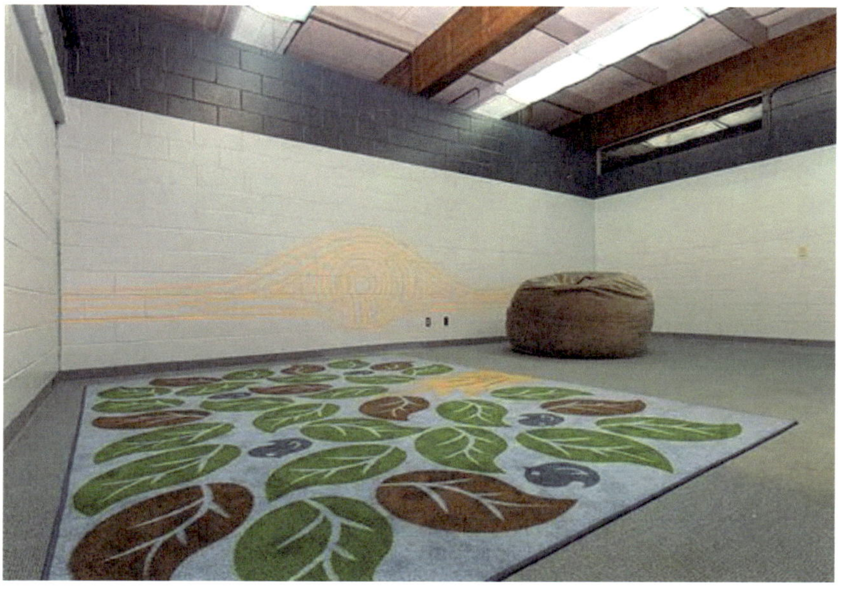

Figure 4.
Finalized Calming Room Space from University of Minnesota Extension (Source: https://bventoumn.wixsite.com/bvento/calmingroom).

Seven themes were identified as follow (1) teachers and staff play a role in helping students calm down, (2) that the use of the calming room supports students in getting back to class sooner, (3) that the calming room has improved the school environment, (4) that students ask to visit the calming room, (5) that the calming room has improved students' self-regulation, (6) that the calming room has increased physical safety, and (7) the importance of simplicity in the calming room design.

2.2.1 Theme 1: Staff help calm

The most prevalent theme (81% of interviews) mentioned in teacher and staff interviews reflected the importance of staff when using the calming room. Even though the calming room was designed with features that promote self-regulation in students, the staff are also an important component to the success of the room:

> *"It gets them back on task again. When they're ready, we can tell and then the students [are] able to talk, you know, we can... process with them a little bit and see what's going on. By the time they go back to the classroom, they're ready."*

The school staff are also important supports that help students stay calm outside of the calming room:

> *"The social workers in our building have been training the entire staff on trauma and how that affects students and what can help students... to self- regulate when they're in the classroom and try and catch on before it escalates."*

Staff also play a role in helping students see and realize that the calming room is a safe space for them – not a place where they are being sent as a punishment:

> *"When they walk into the room, they think they're being isolated... [I say] 'This is just to reset you, to get you back on track.' So in the beginning, you have to explain*

> *to them, 'No, this is not a punishment, this is not a secluded room for you, this is a room that's supposed to be soothing and getting you to know what you're supposed to be doing, getting you back on track."*

These examples provide evidence to the value added by teachers and staff both in the calming room itself and in supporting students' emotion regulation.

2.2.2 Theme 2: Back to class

Another key theme (69% of the interviews) uncovered in the data was that due to the implementation of the calming room, students are returning back to class sooner and more regulated than they did before the calming room was re-designed. One staff member described:

> *"I think it can help kids get back to class faster... whereas before...they did not have that place."*

This outcome is particularly important – if the use of the calming room is leading students to return to the classroom more quickly than before, then they are losing out on less classroom time and can spend more time learning. Students are returning to class more focused and more regulated after having used the calming room:

> *"Once we leave [the calming room], they're more engaged when they go back to the classroom. I think they're more engaged then when they first come into the building in the morning."*

This has also had an impact for students who do not spend time in the calming room, in that their classmates who do use it are returning to class more calm and are less distracting:

> *"It not only helps them, but it also helps the rest of the class so the learning can continue for the other 27 students while that student is calming themselves down, and they come back a lot calmer. ... It's been a lot better than trying to deal with it all in the classroom."*

2.2.3 Theme 3: Improved school environment

The calming room has also benefited the overall school environment (69% of the interviews). Teachers and staff across all types of backgrounds and experiences commented on the reduction in "chaotic movement" in the school. A staff member who spends most time outside of the classrooms reported a notable change in the overall environment:

> *"I know that before the calming room... [it] wasn't as great and it has improved. I can tell that the building is calmer in general."*

Another staff member said, "We don't have as many things being damaged since the room has come into play."

Due to the calming room, students are damaging less and not roaming the halls as much as they did in the past. One staff member even noted the calming effect that the room has had on staff:

> *"I think it's also calming for the staff, I really do. To know that they've got a specifically designed place to take their students, that they're not going to be judged by administration. They're not going to be judged by other staff members... Sometimes if they are going to the library, or the family center it's like 'Oh, they are messing around.'... 'Are they just being allowed to do whatever they want?' But in the calming room, they're not judged there. You take your student there for a specific purpose and you're not judged, so I think it's good for the staff too."*

2.2.4 Theme 4: Students ask

Another theme (69% of the interviews) revealed in the data is that students request to go to the room when they need to calm down. One staff member said: "Some of them have even said, you know, 'I need a break, can I go to that room?". Another staff member reflected upon the usefulness of the calming room for a specific student:

> *"After a while it would seem like he knew that's where he was going so [he would] go and run, he would like run to the room and it's unlocked. And it happened at least once I remember, where he was somewhere in the building... and I found him in there on the bean bag [in the room]."*

Students recognize that the calming room is a positive space they can retreat to when they being to feel dysregulated:

> *"I know that students are being a little more proactive. They're asking to go to the calming room if they kind of starting to get agitated ... they kind of start to get a little agitated or escalating behavior so and they're asking to go there before like: "I just need a break can I go there?" ... It's giving them a tool to kind of regulate their own behavior and you know kind of notice where they are themselves you know some kind of watch themselves."*

Students ask to use the room, willingly take themselves there, and are learning to monitor themselves to know when they should visit it proactively provides evidence that students recognize the value of the calming room.

2.2.5 Theme 5: Emotional regulation

Many of the interviewees reported the room helps students with emotion regulation (63% of interviews). A specially designed space such as the calming room is a key important factor to encouraging students to learn emotional regulation. For example, one respondent said:

> *"The kids seem to be very engaged when they are in there and it does seem to really work its purpose."*

Another staff member commented on the significance of having a room specifically devoted to student emotional regulation rather than a space designed for academic uses:

> *"They stop things from escalating, you know, they gave the student a safe place to go. It wasn't a teacher's office, it wasn't an academic setting per se, so he was able to just go and de-escalate... It's giving them a tool to kind of regulate their own behavior."*

Other staff members also reported how beneficial it was to have a space specifically designed as a calming room:

> *"Before it was there... we would take them to a room and just calm them down but... it didn't have the same calming effect."*

2.2.6 Theme 6: Safety

Teachers and staff reported that the design of the calming room promotes physical safety for students (63% of interviews).

> *"Especially compared to the way it was before the renovation, it's safer now. That's number 1... We're able to just let them be and we don't have to stop them from playing with the sink or go to the pipes or the TV or whatever you know... It's a safer space."*

Interviewees reflected that students are able to express themselves safely in the calming room. One respondent said: "They know it's a safe place." Another component of the theme of safety is that because the students ask to go to the calming room and feel it is safe, staff are less frequently required to use less physical escorts with students:

> *"[Students] are more than willing to walk there without having to be physically escorted."*

The need for fewer physical escorts promotes increased student safety. One teacher commented on the value of having a safe calming room:

> *"I can't imagine not having a safe space like that for when someone gets really dysregulated."*

2.2.7 Theme 7: Simplicity supports regulation

The minimalist, simple design of the calming room is a key facet of its success (25% of interviews). One staff member commented that when a student escalates emotionally they need to "get away from the stimuli." A staff member described the importance of a simple space to promote emotion regulation:

> *"Less is more. So the more things in the room, the more distractions, the more heightened alertness and everything the students already have that they have to deal with."*

A minimalist design also promotes student safety:

> *"[Students] try to find something to break and there's nothing to break, which is great."*

3. Elementary school dining room project

As a result of the positive feedback from the school community about the redesigned Calming room (**Table 1**), the University of Minnesota Extension Children, Youth and Family Consortium initiated another project. This time, the dining hall

Theme	Percentage of sample
Staff help calm	81.25%
Back to class	68.75%
Improved school environment	68.75%
Students ask	68.75%
Emotional regulation	62.5%
Safety	62.5%
Importance of simplicity	25.0%

Table 1.
Themes related to the calming room (n = 16).

at Bruce Vento became the venue for renovation. An undergraduate Interior design student collaborated with the first author in a funded undergraduate research project to develop design solutions for the dining space taking into account the need for a healthy eating and trauma-sensitive space [16]. The project goal was to reduce the noise level and address circulation issues in the existing dining space. The original dining hall's loud eating environment, institutional atmosphere, and a limited amount of natural light contributed to a sterile environment (**Figure 5**). These characteristics can negatively impact disruptive behavior especially in students with behavioral challenges. The University of Minnesota Extension Children, Youth and Family Consortium staff, interior design team (author 1 and interior design student), and the Bruce Vento team explored best practices to have a positive impact on the dining hall at the school and toured the design spaces of a leading edge school, the Creative Arts School in St. Paul to study best practices and gain inspiration.

3.1 The design

To create a welcoming and nurturing dining environment to foster students' learning and to support their health several ideas emerged from research, ideation and team brainstorming. The ideas included creating a teaching kitchen space for nutrition educators to use with students and families, promoting family dining style

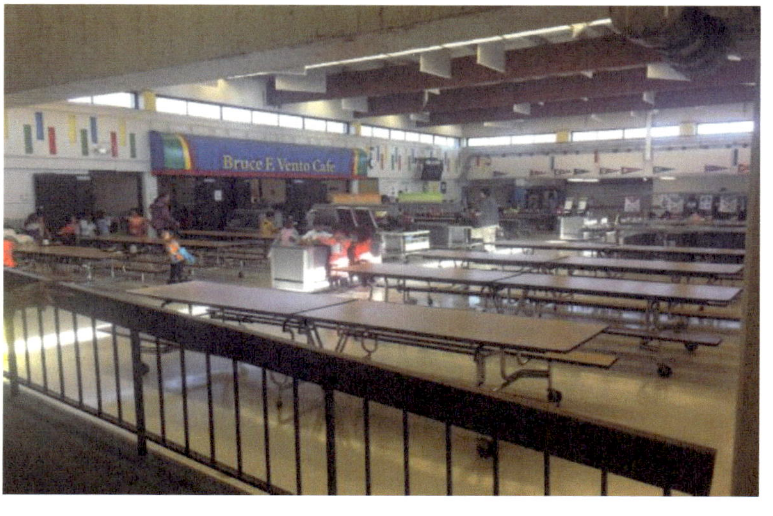

Figure 5.
Bruce Vento dining hall former Interior condition. (Source: Picture by Author 1)

and healthy eating through round tables, and solving acoustical problems by adding sound absorbing materials in the dining space (**Figure 6**). Recognizing there is no simple solution and "one size does not fit all," the team prioritized six design solutions (**Figure 7**): (1) sound reduction materials, (2) family style eating to increase times for eating, (3) natural elements create calming and restorative environment, (4) teaching spaces for students and parents, (5) communal eating spaces, and (6) glass walls that provide light and open feeling. However, due to the financial restriction, the team was only able to implement a design that reduced noise levels and enabled positive interactions. The team focused on one major change, which is a shift from long, rectangular tables to round tables (**Figure 8**). The round tables were funded through an internal grant received from the University of Minnesota by Author 1.

3.2 Evaluation

As mentioned earlier, the team was able to only change one major thing, the furniture which is a change from long and rectangular tables to round tables. One small change was enough to make a big difference. In the new layout, condiments, napkins, and utensils were placed in the center of each table, based on dining room workers' input. This placement reduced noise levels dramatically because students did not need to get up and retrieve condiments or utensils from the other end of a long table. Both the dining hall workers and students noticed the change and liked it. In a quieter and calmer dining hall, students' stress levels may decrease and they are making better food choices and having richer interactions with their friends. A 5th grader told 5abc Eyewitness News, in an interview regarding the design intervention at Bruce Vento elementary school, "Last year it was very loud, and this is a little bit more quiet... when nothing is loud, it is all peaceful" [17].

The teachers' feedback on the dining hall renovation was also positive. 91% of the teachers surveyed preferred the new round tables in the dining hall. The teachers reported the round table, above all, created senses of "inclusivity" and family style dining which encouraged students to interact and socialize while staying

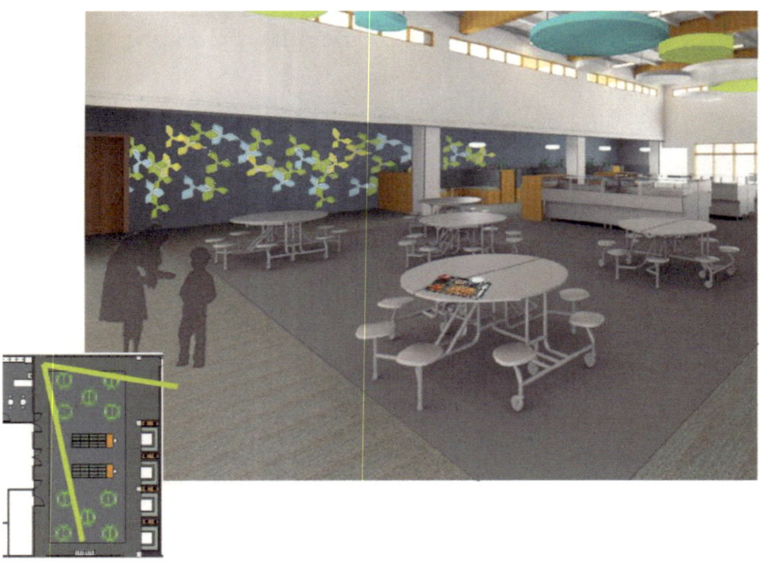

Figure 6.
Bruce Vento dining hall schematic design. (Source: Rendering by Miranda McNamara).

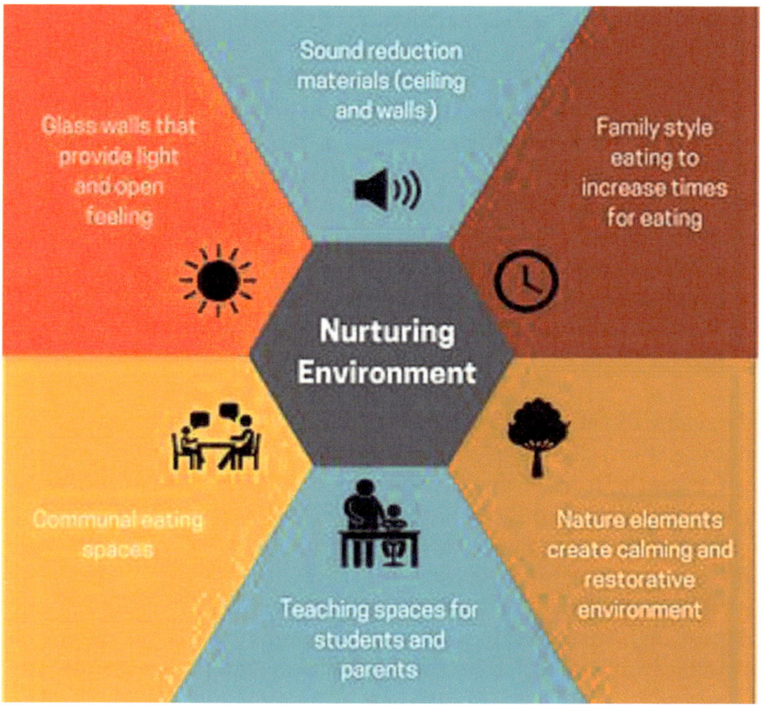

Figure 7.
Six prioritized design solutions for Bruce Vento dining hall redesign (Source: https://bventoumn.wixsite.com/bvento/calmingroom).

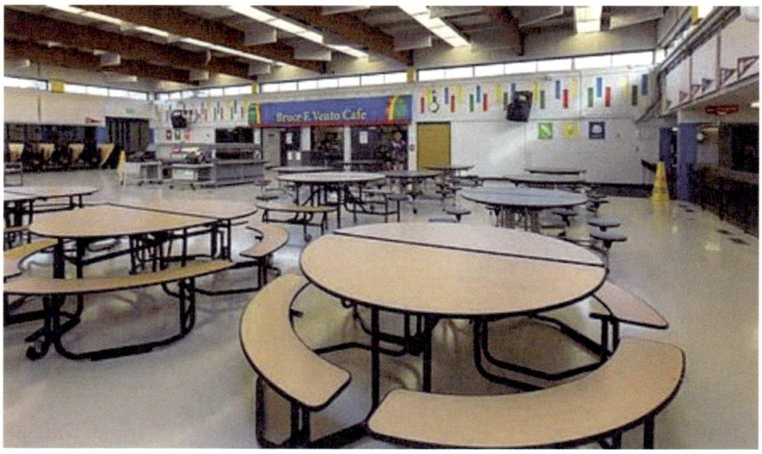

Figure 8.
Finished condition of Bruce Vento dining hall with the round tables (Source: https://bventoumn.wixsite.com/bvento/calmingroom).

seated. As the staff observed, the dining hall became less "institutional" and more "communal" which turned the overall atmosphere into "kinder" and "gentler". Suggestions for future improvements of the dining hall include "adding more components to contribute more to the family feel", adjusting current lighting conditions (e.g., "too harsh", "lower light", etc.), and providing wall storages to optimize student circulations.

4. Elementary school teacher sanctuary project

Both the calming room and dining hall contributed to the healthy development of elementary students in Bruce Vento School. These benefits of the new environments had to be extended to the school resource staff and teachers. As influencers who make significant differences in student success, teachers and school staff need the time and space to recharge and refuel for their important job of leading children's development. This led our interdisciplinary team and the school to collaborate on renovating the current teacher lounge (**Figure 9**). The goal of the space was to accommodate the needs of teachers, paraprofessionals, and other support staff during the day [18].

4.1 The design

As the first step of the design process, a need-analysis was conducted by engaging teachers to understand their expectations and necessities. The need analysis involved a wide range of methods including face-to-face conversation, in an online survey, and in an informal focus group in their lounge space. Throughout the processes, the team learned that the current lounge was not used frequently by many teachers due to several reasons (e.g., not an appealing environment, not properly functional amenities like the sink and cupboards, and lacked a sense of permanence with frequent changes in physical location). Based on these current problems and the teachers' needs, three guiding principles and strategies for the new teacher sanctuary were defined: (1) start small, and add more later; (2) build for multiple uses: community, relaxation, eating, and refueling; and (3) accommodate both teachers and teaching support staff.

> *"Relaxing lighting, comfortable seating, food preparation [space],[piped-in] music, wall decorations, [a] staff kudos board, places for information to share with staff. So much opportunity!"*

Within the three guiding principles, the team took several considerations for the project: (1) infusing natural light through lamps; (2) creating distinct spaces with

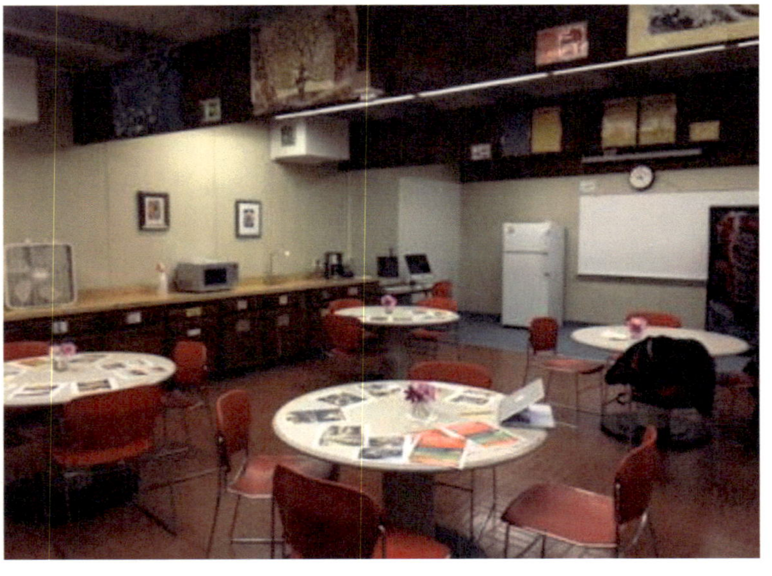

Figure 9.
Bruce Vento teacher lounge former Interior condition. (Source: Picture by Author 1)

partitions; (3) adding a communal table to facilitate communications; (4) maintaining computers in the room for staff needs; (5) creating ample space for meal prep and easy clean up; and (6) improving overall appeal with colored walls and few, but high impact design touches.

After a year, the project was completed during the summer break in 2017. **Figure 10** offers a comprehensive timeline description of the design and implementation process from start to finish. The final solution features a straightforward and functional layout. A central interactive area was a major portion of the space and it opened opportunities for collaborations and communications between teachers, staff and related personnel. At one end of the room, the relaxation space provides a location where teachers sit down and rejuvenate their energy plus motivation (**Figure 11**). For the implementation, Room and Board, a home décor retailer in Golden Valley Minnesota, inspired by the project and its purpose donated furniture to implement the proposed design at the school (**Figure 12**).

4.2 Evaluation

The school staff and teachers started using the completed space in summer 2017. The design, layout, and overall environment of the new space was different from the previous teacher's lounge. The school started to stock the cupboards with staple items, utensils, and extra coffee machines. According to the feedback from the teachers, they were satisfied with the new space which aligned with the initial project objectives. The teacher sanctuary, like all the initiatives undertaken at Bruce Vento Elementary School, will continue to evolve as users' needs and circumstances change.

After the project, an interview was conducted to learn how the teachers think about the new space. The teachers, especially, thought the redesigned space supports their well-being because it is relaxing with soothing colors, gives peaceful energy to recharge, and provides a comfortable place to get away. They also perceived the new space as welcoming and inviting space to meet their colleagues. There was a comment about cleanliness. The tables are not as dirty as they used to be, and that may be because the attractiveness inspires people to clean up after themselves. One teacher, in particular, mentioned that they used the space as an area to regroup and

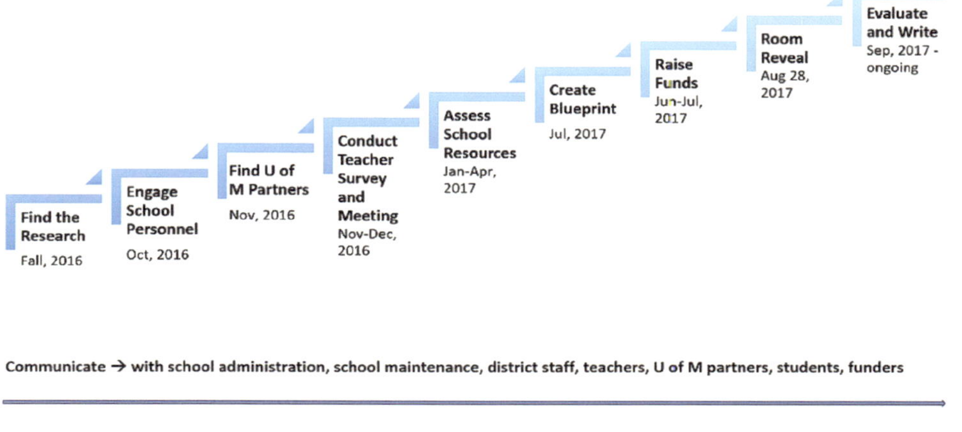

Figure 10.
The design and implementation process of Bruce Vento teacher sanctuary from 2016 to 2017. The steps are finding the research, engaging school personnel, finding U of M partners, conducting teacher survey and meeting, assessing school resources, creating blueprint, raising fund, revealing room, and ongoing reflection (Source: https://bventoumn.wixsite.com/bvento/calmingroom).

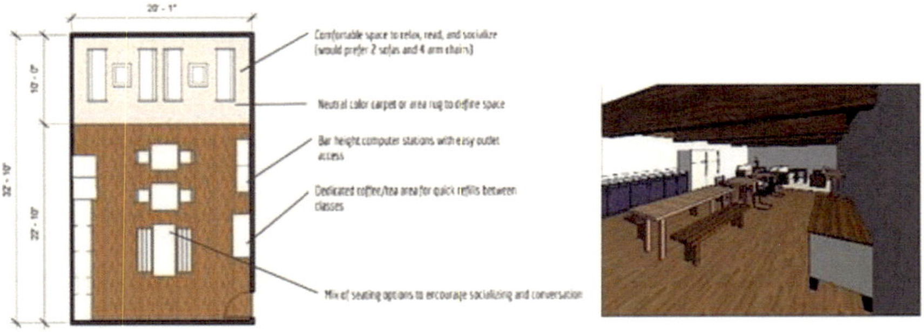

Figure 11.
The Bruce Vento teacher sanctuary proposed design (Source: Drawings by Noah Exum and Abigail Lundstrom).

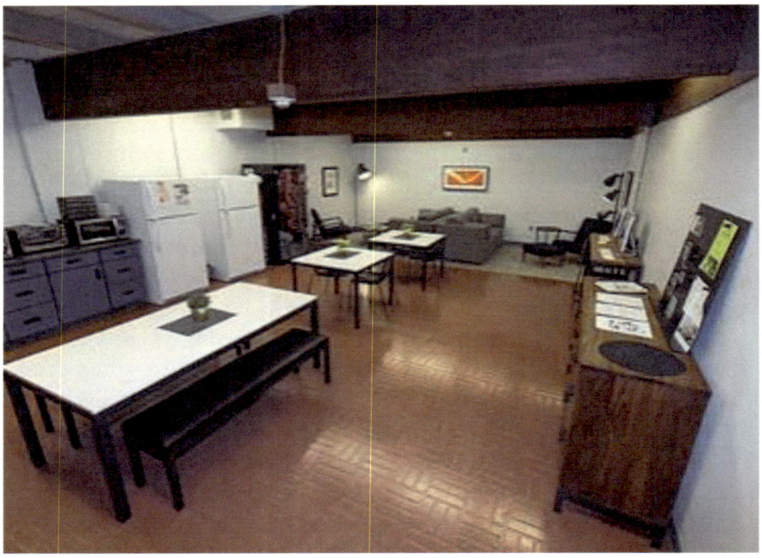

Figure 12.
The renovation of Teacher sanctuary space (Source: https://bventoumn.wixsite.com/bvento/calmingroom).

refocus after helping students that are having a hard time. Therefore, there is no doubt that people use the new space to refresh themselves and like the space.

In addition, the teachers also thought the new space supports community building for school staff, mainly because they use the space for various purposes. They used the space as a gathering place, and they liked to see more people in the space, as the space is bigger than the previous staff lounge. In addition, they have a bi-weekly staff treat in the space. The teachers mentioned that as the space has plenty of room to have a nice spread of food, many utensils and supplies, it is a great place to accommodate many staff at once. One teacher said that food is set out in the new lounge, and different staff eat together in the lounge. Another teacher also mentioned that the new space is very nice for substitute teachers to eat or relax during prep time. Based on the teachers' responses, they appreciated the spacious and relaxing space for them.

> *"It's a welcoming, calm environment that provides some solace in the midst of a sometimes challenging day. [The new space supports staff community-building because] there's more people, more connections, and higher morale."*

DOI: http://dx.doi.org/10.5772/intechopen.97525

5. Conclusion

Findings from the teacher and staff interviews support the literature about the impact of calming rooms and dining spaces in supporting students' emotional and self-regulation at the Bruce Vento School environment. There was an overall improved environment in the school, likely because students are able to regulate themselves and are asking to go use the calming room – a safe space where they can get the support they need and return to class. The new space allows staff to support and help students learn how to self-regulate, calm down, and then return to class sooner than before the space was redesigned. As in previous studies [9], students at the school ask to visit the calming room and recognize that it is a dedicated space where they can retreat to and feel safe. Also mirroring previous efforts in non-school settings, the implementation of the calming room leads to reductions in the amount of physical restraints staff had to use with students [19–21], thus increasing student safety. The data reinforced the strengths of approaching design problem solving through partnerships that seek out multiple perspectives. The simplicity of the final design solution implemented resulted from engaging multiple perspectives through interview of the clients, site visit, research, presentation, and feedback from clients. Likewise, the school community reported the new dining space created an inclusive and communal family style dining environment [22–27]. The round family style dining tables reduced students' traffic and movement to retrieve condiments or utensils from the other end of a long table and this reduced the noise level in the dining space. The school staff observed the family style dining encouraged interaction and socialization among students and the dining space became less institutional and more communal. Additionally, the new teacher sanctuary extended the benefits of the new environment to the school resource staff and teachers. The teacher sanctuary created a space for school staff to rejuvenate and to help support their job of leading children's development [28–30].

Finally, through this collaborative process, interior design students gained disciplinary and civic benefits such as application of their course knowledge, opportunities to connect to the community through real life design issues. The opportunity to visit the existing space and tour with the users to gather information and experience the space physically gave students better understanding of the space, building systems, and requirements for the projects. Overall, all the three design projects led to positive outcomes for the school community. Through the partnership with Bruce Vento Elementary School, a calming room, teacher sanctuary, and family style dining hall were all implemented in the school to build community and create a trauma sensitive environment. Anecdotal evidence shows that this Bruce Vento community building model of creating a trauma sensitive environment that fosters health and well-being has been used as a precedent for other school districts in Minneapolis St Paul.

Author details

Abimbola O. Asojo[1*], Hoa Vo[1], Suyeon Bae[2], Chelsea Hetherington[3], Sarah Cronin[4] and Judy Myers[5]

1 University of Minnesota, College of Design, St. Paul, Minnesota, USA

2 Architectural Studies, University of Missouri, Columbia, Missouri, USA

3 Department of Human Development and Family Studies, University of Illinois at Urbana-Champaign, Urbana, Illinois, USA

4 Psychology Department, Bemidji State University, Bemidji, Minnesota, USA

5 UMN Extension Children, Youth and Family Consortium, University of Minnesota, St. Paul, Minnesota, USA

*Address all correspondence to: aasojo@umn.edu

References

[1] Boston D, Ross B, Weglarz P. Playful Thursday project: Community/ university partners and lessons learned in a longitudinal study. J Community Engagement Scholarship. 2017;10(1):13.

[2] Casapulla S, Hess ME. Engagement education: A model of community-youth engagement in rural Appalachia. J Community Engagement Scholarship. 2017;9(2):5.

[3] Burrell S. Trauma and the environment of care in juvenile institutions. Retrieved Sept. 2013;9:2014.

[4] Fraser K, MacKenzie D, Versnel J. Complex trauma in children and youth: A scoping review of sensory-based interventions. Occup Ther Ment Heal. 2017;33(3):199-216.

[5] Renwick F, Spalding B. Research Section:'A Quiet Place'Project: an of Early Therapeutic Intervention within Mainstream Schools. British Journal of Special Education. 2002 Sep;29(3): 144-50.

[6] Blackburn, R. Many parents and pros advocating 'calming rooms' for schools [Internet]. Athens Banner Herald. 2010 [cited 2021Mar31]. Available from: http://onlineathens.com/stories/051110/ new_637263838.shtml/#.WgYVwTBry70

[7] Chagaris C. How to Design a Calming Room for Autistic Kids [Internet]. 2015 [cited 2021 Jan 2]. Available from: http://www.nymetroparents.com/ article/How-To-Design-a-Calming-Room-for-Autistic-Kids

[8] Moore K. Sensory Room for adults or adolescents in mental health setting [Internet]. The Sensory Connection program. [cited 2021Mar31]. Available from: http://www. sensoryconnectionprogram.com/ sensory_room.php

[9] King A, Chantler Z. Focus on Practice: The Western Primary School 'Quiet Room 'Project. Br J Spec Educ. 2002;29(4):183-8.

[10] Evans GW, Kim P. Childhood poverty, chronic stress, self-regulation, and coping. Child Dev Perspect. 2013;7(1):43-8.

[11] Peter Kraftl. Environment for children: passive lessons from the everyday environment. Children's Geographies. 2008; 6:1: 109-110, DOI: 10.1080/14733280701791983

[12] Brown J. A school's dining environment: Why is it Important? [Internet]. 2010 [cited 2021 Jan 2]. Available from: https://www.ecoliteracy. org/article/school's-dining-environment-why-it-important

[13] MacDaniel, M., Van Bramer, J., Hogan, M. F. Comfort rooms: A preventative tool used to reduce the use of restraint and seclusion in facilities that serve individuals with mental illness [Internet]. New York State's Office of Mental Health. n.d. [cited 2021Mar31]. Available from: https:// omh.ny.gov/omhweb/resources/ publications/comfort_room/comfort_ rooms.pdf

[14] Hydon S, Wong M, Langley AK, Stein BD, Kataoka SH. Preventing secondary traumatic stress in educators. Child and Adolescent Psychiatric Clinics. 2015 Apr 1;24(2):319-33.

[15] The University of Minnesota Extension Children, Youth & Family. Calming Room [Internet]. Bruce Vento University of Minnesota. 2015 [cited 2021Mar31]. Available from: https:// bventoumn.wixsite.com/bvento/ calmingroom

[16] The University of Minnesota Extension Children, Youth & Family.

The Dining Hall [Internet]. Bruce Vento University of Minnesota. 2015 [cited 2021Mar31]. Available from: https://bventoumn.wixsite.com/bvento/dininghall

[17] Eyewitness News. Can Design Changes Lead To Mood Changes? St. Paul Elementary School To Find Out [Internet]. KSTP. 2017 [cited 2021Mar31]. Available from: from http://kstp.com/news/mood-changes-design-changes-st-paul-elementary/4609159/

[18] The University of Minnesota Extension Children, Youth & Family. Teacher Sanctuary [Internet]. Bruce Vento University of Minnesota. 2015 [cited 2021Mar31]. Available from: https://bventoumn.wixsite.com/bvento/teachersanctuary

[19] Bobier C, Boon T, Downward M, Loomes B, Mountford H, Swadi H. Pilot investigation of the use and usefulness of a sensory modulation room in a child and adolescent psychiatric inpatient unit. Occup Ther Ment Heal. 2015;31(4):385-401.

[20] Warner E, Koomar J, Lary B, Cook A. Can the body change the score? Application of sensory modulation principles in the treatment of traumatized adolescents in residential settings. J Fam Violence. 2013;28(7): 729-38.

[21] Asojo AO, Patel T. Community Participatory Design Process for an Autism Clinic: Role+ Pedagogy+ Reflection. Journal of Interior Design. In: Proceedings of the 2017 EDRA48 Madison Annual Conference. 31 May- 3 June 2017; Madison. p.157-163.

[22] Brown, J. A school's dining environment: Why is it Important? [Internet]. Ecoliteracy. 2010 [cited 2021Mar31]. Available from: https://www.ecoliteracy.org/article/school%E2%80%99s-dining-environment-why-it-important

[23] Gage, L. Recreating school cafeterias: A menu of creative options [Internet]. Global Educator Institute. 2015 [cited 2021Mar31]. Available from: http://bit.ly/2kHbcFs

[24] Health Promotion Agency for Northern Ireland. Improving the dining experience in schools [Internet]. Public Health. n.d. [cited 2021Mar31]. Available from: http://www.publichealth.hscni.net/sites/default/files/Dining%20Experience%2009_10.pdf

[25] Kuong, P. Redesigning the school cafeteria [Internet]. HuffPost. 2013 [cited 2021Mar31]. Available from: http://bit.ly/2zgpvnC

[26] The School Food Plan. Tips on improving the dining experience [Internet]. What Works Well. 2014 [cited 2021Mar31]. Available from: http://bit.ly/2zgkBXy

[27] Wansin, B., Just, D. R., McKendry, J. Lunch line redesign [Internet]. The New York Times. 2010 [cited 2021Mar31]. Available from: http://nyti.ms/1NrTs5b

[28] Ben-Peretz M, Schonmann S, Kupermintz H. The teachers' lounge and its role in improving learning environments in schools. School climate: Measuring, improving, and sustaining healthy learning environments. 1999 Apr 1:148e164.

[29] Mawhinney L. Let's lunch and learn: Professional knowledge sharing in teachers' lounges and other congregational spaces. Teaching and Teacher Education. 2010 May 1;26(4):972-8.

[30] Shapiro S. Revisiting the teachers' lounge: Reflections on emotional experience and teacher identity. Teaching and teacher education. 2010 Apr 1;26(3):616-21.

Chapter 8

Surgical Outpatient Care: Triage, Time and Test

Satyendra K. Tiwary

Abstract

Day care surgery is the standard of care for minor surgical procedures in developed countries and rapidly increasing in practice in developing countries. The main advantages of day care surgery are cost containment, early mobilization of the patient, less pain because of minimally invasive surgical techniques, early return of patient to their home and work. The downsides of day care surgery include the inability to treat all patients and perform all surgical procedures since surgical fitness for day care procedures is demanding, unforeseen readmission, the need for more operating rooms, and increasing expertise among health care workers. Considering day care surgery as systematic, scheduled and short duration stay in hospital, it is very important to select or sort out the cases which fit in the criteria according to all conventional definitions of triage. It is well organized within stipulated time frame and performed in fixed unit with proper assessment by anesthesia and nursing team in addition to core assessment of surgical team. Surgical option exercised and close follow up with ability to manage complications are integral components in working team. Delivery of more surgery in primary care has potential for enhancing patient-centred management by promoting the development of multi-specialty community providers and reducing length of hospital stay. The outpatient surgical centers provide many benefits and advantages for surgical patients with proper organizations, dedicated services, and meticulous procedures.

Keywords: Day Care Surgery, Outpatient Surgery, Anesthesia, Day care set up

1. Introduction

Day care surgery is the standard of care for minor surgical procedures in developed countries and rapidly increasing in practice in developing countries. It is a rapidly evolving and widely accepted way of catering health care to the masses [1]. Patients were in the past, customarily admitted to hospital for all but the most trivial of surgical operations and remained until they are self-sufficient, ambulant and their sutures removed Considered obligatory for wound healing, post-operative bed rest up to 21 days was commonly enforced on patients in the past [2].

The main advantages of day surgery are cost control, early patient activity, less pain caused by minimally invasive surgical techniques, early return of patients to the home environment, reduced risk of cross-infection in the hospital, and fewer wage losses due to early return. Under the background of making good use of resources, due to the advancement of anesthesia technology and the development of surgical technology, you can quickly and smoothly resume work [3]. The disadvantage of day care surgery is that it cannot be performed on all patients and all surgical operations, because day care surgery requires high surgical applicability, unexpected readmissions, more operating rooms, and higher skills of health personnel.

Commonly used day care procedures (**Tables 1** and **2**) settings include hydrocele, hernia, varicose veins, varicocele, anal fissure, breast tumor resection, and diagnostic laparoscopic surgery. Hernia is one of the common surgical problems in daily practice in developing countries [1]. It constitutes the majority of waiting cases before surgery in outpatient surgery departments, especially in government hospitals. The postoperative bed occupancy rate of these patients is also very high, making it difficult to rationally use beds in public hospitals In public hospitals, even for important cases such as malignant tumors, the waiting period for intervention is very long.

Day care surgery can shorten the waiting list and help rationalize the cost of surgical treatment. Hence, the demand for day care surgeries in India is increasing. Although its advantages are widely used in developed countries, the rate of use in developing countries is very low. There are many factors that affect the success of day care surgery, such as the financial limitations of developing independent day-care units, inadequate primary health care facilities, and the psychosocial factors of the patients.

General surgery	Gynecology	Trauma	Maxillofacial
Incision and drainage of abscess	Evacuation of retained products of conception	Tendon repair	MUA fractured nose
Laparoscopic cholecystectomy	Laparoscopic ectopic pregnancy	MUA of fracture	Repair of fractured mandible
Laparoscopic appendicectomy		Plating of fractured bone	
Temporal artery biopsy			

Table 1.
Types of urgent surgery suitable for day case procedures.

Breast surgery	Excision of breast
	Simple mastectomy
	Sentinal node biopsy
	Axillary clearance
Gynecology	Operations to manage female incontinence
Urology	Endoscopic resection of prostate (TURP)
	Resection of prostate by laser
General surgery	Cholecystectomy
	Repair of a range of hernia
Orthopedic surgery	Arthoscopic subacromial decompression
	Bunion operations
	Dupuytren's fasciectomy
ENT	Tympanoplasty
	Tonsillectomy
	Septoplasty

Table 2.
Commonly performed day care surgery.

DOI: http://dx.doi.org/10.5772/intechopen.100170

The factors associated with the success of outpatient surgery are adequate patient selection, adequate patient information, preoperative evaluation, anesthesia and good postoperative analgesia, patient acceptance, and effective review. The concept of day care surgery helps reduce these problems by facilitating early discharge of patients undergoing minor surgery. This concept has been widely accepted by developed countries because their socio-economic status and medical and healthcare facilities are very good. Inguinal hernia is one of the most common surgical problems, but because the development of hernia involves complex anatomy and pathology, it still confuses surgeons.

2. Triage in day care surgery

Considering the day care surgery as systematic, scheduled and short duration stay in hospital, it is very important to select or sort out the cases which fit in the criteria according to all conventional definitions of triage. It is well organized within stipulated time frame and performed in fixed unit with proper assessment by anesthesia and nursing team in addition to core assessment of surgical team. Surgical option exercised and close follow up with ability to manage complications are integral components in working team. So, considering the all the components of Day Care Surgery (DCS), it is very important to try to sort out the cases according to priority, feasibility, associated risks, outcomes and follow-up. Every factor should be considered in anesthetic and nursing team check selected for day care surgery must be thoroughly and completely examined by anesthesia and nursing team. Once anesthetics checkup and nursing evaluation is complete, surgeries are planned and those cases who are not fit in Day Care surgery must be sent or referred back to the corresponding unit for proper management. After selection of the cases, adequate and complete evaluations are must before putting them for surgery and after surgery this should be evaluated again, advised again with key focus for early identification of postoperative complications and management. Patient is advised to report, call or come back earliest so communication is quite important in cases of Day Care surgery as compared to others. Triage of cases in for day care surgery can be divided into three types of patients:

1. **Selected:** Those cases who are selected for the day care surgery with all pre requisite and criteria fulfilled (ASA I & II).

2. **Selected but** special **care needed:** In ASA III, usually day care surgery not advised but with special care and close follow up with extended recovery protocol.

3. **Not selected:** Those who are not in the category of Day Care surgery are sent back or referred.

3. Success, surgery and selection

Success story for day surgery always includes patient selection, operation selection, surgeon qualification, nurse qualification, and team construction and management.

Patient's fitness for day surgery should be judged by functional assessment just before preoperative assessment. There are few medical conditions once fully optimized which would exclude a patient from day surgery.

3.1 Patient selection

Patients must have adequate family and social support, especially in the first 24 hours after surgery. The patient must use transportation within 24 hours after the operation. You can take a private car driven by a driver other than the patient, or you can use a 24-hour taxi service. They must live within a two-hour drive from the hospital. The selection of outpatient surgery patients is also based on their general health and age. After completing the practice, the following basic requirements are put forward to the patient:

1. **American Association of Anesthesiologists (ASA) Scale**: Generally speaking, only ASA I and II patients are eligible for normal day surgery. It should be noted that there is literature on ASA III patients undergoing outpatient surgery, with a low complication rate [3, 4].

2. **Age:** The literature shows that outpatient surgery has been successfully completed and is suitable for patients of all ages. For example, patients older than 1 year undergo pediatric surgery, patients under 60 years old undergo laparoscopic cholecystectomy (LC) in adults, and the cut-off age for varicose vein and hernia repair is less than 70 years [5].

3. **Body Mass Index (BMI):** Being overweight or obese will increase the difficulty and incidence of postoperative complications. Hypertension, congestive heart failure, and snoring are the main postoperative complications associated with obese patients [3]. British guidelines for outpatient surgery stipulate that patients with a BMI of 35 kg / m2 can receive outpatient surgery if they are fully optimized [3, 6].

4. **Co-morbidities** associated**:** Chronic diseases are not contraindications to surgery and can be included in day surgery as long they are stable and non-progressive, known to the anesthesiologists and surgeons. Examples include hypertension, diabetes, and coronary artery atherosclerotic heart disease. However, end-stage diseases such as liver failure, congestive cardiac failure and kidney failure are excluded from day care surgery [7].

3.2 Surgical option and selection

A list of surgery approved and developed by the Surgical Management Committee during the day must be obtained. The standard is as follows.

a. Estimated operating time of less than 2 hours (which allows you to walk early and promote fast recovery),

b. Management of postoperative pain due to the formulation of oral analgesic drugs, and

c. There is no special postoperative care for the hometown.

3.3 Surgical expertise

Surgeons must be enthusiastic and committed to the development of day care surgery. Senior consultants with experience over 10 years with the ability to operate independently and have completed a minimum number of cases.

3.4 Nursing parameter

Nurses must have a minimum of 10 years of expertise in managing pre- and post-operative care with proper communication skills, vast knowledge in different disciplines, and knowledge of rules in hospital, national health policies, and medical bill reimbursement procedures with insurance coverage [3].

4. Day care set up

Day-care surgery should ideally be provided in a self-contained unit that is functionally and structurally separate from inpatient wards and theaters. The possible suggestion for such functioning may involve [8, 9].

4.1 Hospital integrated

Ambulatory surgical patients are managed in the same surgery facility as inpatients. Outpatients may have separate preoperative preparation and recovery areas.

4.2 Hospital based

A separate ambulatory surgical facility within a hospital handles only outpatients.

4.3 Free standing

These surgical and diagnostic facilities may be associated with a hospital or medical center but are housed in separate buildings that share no space or patient care functions. Preoperative evaluation, surgical care, and recovery occur within these autonomic units. In developing nations, majority of nursing homes and smaller hospitals function in this manner.

4.4 Office based

These operating or diagnostic units are managed in conjunction with physician's offices for the convenience of patients and health-care providers.

5. Eligibility criteria for day care surgery

Screening, selection and surgery of the patients requires certain fixed eligibility criteria and that should be followed meticulously and methodically which is summarized as [9]:

- Patient must be sound to understand the delicate intricacies of day-care procedures.
- During discharge from hospital, an adult person should accompany the patient with written instructions.
- The domestic environment should be conducive enough for smooth postoperative period.

- Besides evaluating basic minimum laboratory investigations, clinical acumen is very important in deciding the fitness for day-care surgery and anesthesia.
- Comorbid diseases should be optimized satisfactorily before declaring patient fit for surgery.
- Decision of day-care surgical procedures also depends on the duration, severity, and potential chances of hemodynamic instability and others.
- Patient should be able to initiate oral intake within few hours of the surgical procedure.
- Anesthetic drugs and techniques should be chosen in manner not to disturb the postoperative ambulation.
- Patient should be able to take care of himself/herself for routine personal chores.
- A good means of transport and communication should be available to the patient at home.
- Availability of physician/surgeon for 24 h is an essential prerequisite in case of any emergency readmission.

5.1 Advantages of outpatient surgery

There are many advantages of outpatient surgery which have an edge over traditional, inpatient surgical procedures. These include the following [8, 10, 11]:

A. **Convenience.** The convenience of recovering in your home generally makes recovery time faster than an in-hospital stay.

B. **Cost effective.** Since there are many aspects including hospital room charges, and associated hospital charges which are curtailed in outpatient surgery leading to cost effectiveness and reduced cost in the treatment. Some surgical procedures are covered in health insurance only on an outpatient basis which may be under the umbrella of day care surgery.

C. **Less stress.** Outpatient surgery leads to less stress on surgical team in the majority of cases, inpatient surgery. Most people prefer to stay in hospital less and less and better for them to recover in their homes rather than in the hospital.

D. **Well Scheduled.** In a hospital setting, first priority are emergency surgeries and procedures which can be unpredictable in outcome and volume and that can delay the scheduled surgeries. In such situations, an outpatient setting can generally stay within a set schedule since the procedures are less complex and more routine.

E. **Reduced hospital infections.** Due to shorter hospital stay and meticulous, timely work plan, incidence of nosocomial infections is reduced markedly. A significant post-operative morbidity in the form of hospital acquired infections is reduced leading to patient satisfaction and less economic burden with smooth functions in post-operative phase.

F. **Efficiency.** Shorter waiting list for surgery, less hospital bed occupancy, more surgery, flexibility due to non-dependency on hospital beds leads to increased efficiency of the system leading to increased number of surgeries for any hospital set up.

5.2 Disadvantages of outpatient surgery

However, day-care anesthesia and surgery are associated with certain limitations and disadvantages which include but are not limited to the following [8, 10, 11]:

A. **Complications:** Surgical and anesthetic complications are relatively a stress resulting in unplanned admissions once there is any post-operative major complications.

B. **Expertise:** A higher expertise level is required in day care surgery for providing results in timely, organized and planned way as compared to routine surgery admissions.

C. **Pre-anesthetic lacunae:** It is always a possibility of missing the important points in pre-operative anesthetic checkup and possible chances of negligence may be increased.

D. **Compliance:** There might be poor compliance from the patients regarding medications, instructions about fasting and post-operative protocol after discharge as they are not admitted for the long duration to remain under supervision.

E. **Anxiety:** Level of anxiety is more in day care surgery in more apprehensive patients as they are worried more about short hospital stay.

5.3 Contra-indications of outpatient surgery

It is not advisable always for outpatient surgery as there are certain limitations which must be considered. Uncontrolled hypertension, severe respiratory disorders, smoking, obesity is considered the major contraindications for daycare surgery. The surgeons often suggest such patients go for elective surgeries which is better in such high-risk patients. In any kind of surgery, such patients will be recovered in a better way without confronting any of the complications. Whether it is a traditional or elective or a daycare surgery, proper care should be taken for such patients. Meticulous assessment to rule out significant co-morbidity is the key factor for excluding the cases unfit for the day care surgery.

6. Protocol in day care surgery

Day care surgery follows standard and set protocols which have been formulated and followed globally [12]. First and foremost, point is pre anesthetic assessment and preparation according to protocol driven nurse-led discharge in each and every patient. This is the key principle in day care surgery patients. Day care surgery patients are mostly from outpatient clinics, sometimes from emergency departments or satellite care or primary care centres. Technical advancements in surgery, anesthesia and investigations have set the momentum for day care surgery globally and many surgical procedures are being performed but protocols must be followed for every procedure. Social, medical and surgical assessment of every patient coming for day care surgery should be included and multidisciplinary approach mast be followed with inclusion and exclusion criteria set before. Planned procedure must the explained to the patient before surgery, post-operative care explained and advice with collaboration with the nursing team in preoperative preparation. Three components must be emphasized which includes education and care explained to the patient regarding surgical intervention, information about planned procedures and post-operative care with informed decisions and documented important information to identify medical risk factors, promote health and optimized patients' conditions. Three components well explained which are essential and must include all three teams of surgery, anesthesia and nursing so day care surgery had in its protocol with three teams and under three headings of time, triage and test with three components well summarized again:

1. Education and care explained to the patient regarding surgical intervention,

2. Information about planned procedures and post-operative care with informed decisions

3. Documented important information to identify medical risk factors, promote health and optimized patients' conditions

7. Tests and practices in day care surgery

Definite set of procedures are always performed and in practice as per pathology present in the patient. Blood investigations and biopsy are two tests that are helping to decide the underlying inflammatory or malignant condition. Apart from imaging in radiology (X ray/USG/CT/MRI/Mammogram) endoscopy and endoscopic USG are integral tests for diagnosis in hollow viscera pathology. Majority of the day care surgery are breast surgery and biopsy with mammogram needed in almost all cases. With continuous evolution in endoscopy, it is endoscopic USG which may detect the underlying pathology close to any hollow viscera and even guided FNAC may yield the diagnosis. Tests to be done depending upon underlying pathology can be summarized as

- Blood tests
- X-rays
- Ultrasound
- CT/MRI Scan
- Mammograms
- Pan endoscopy
- Endoscopic USG
- Biopsy

8. Core issues and key points

The operational system should include the following summary points to clear the management of certain key issues. These include:

1. Screening and selection of the patients with proper history, examination and scrutiny of medical records.

2. Surgical option must be tailored as per the requirement.

3. Pre-anesthetic checkup, and examination by nursing care team should be done before surgery

4. Proper system of medical emergencies in the adverse events of cardiac arrest, major hemorrhage, respiratory distress preferably in the same set up and the availability of equipment, drugs and skilled personnel to manage the complications with the hemorrhage availability of anesthesia team back up always.

5. Robust, tested, clear communications and written service level transfer agreements between the stand-alone unit, the nearest acute hospital, its intensive care unit and the ambulance service.

6. Management of patients who cannot be discharged home or something unpredictable event preventing discharge.

7. Management of patients with complications with proper communications following the discharge (**Table 3**).

8. There should be clear information and complete communication provided to patients as to where to go if complications occur.

9. Appropriate cover advised until patients are discharged from the hospital

10. Teaching, training, supervision and opportunities for research and future planning

11. Regular audit and analysis of the services provided to detect and sort out the lacunae to improve overall the service and results.

• The patient is alert and able to adapt to time, place and person
• Stable vital signs
• Oral analgesics control pain
• Controlled nausea and vomiting
• Able to walk without accidents
• No bleeding at the surgical site
• Receipt of discharge instructions and prescription
• Patient accepts preparation for discharge
• Person in charge of escort

Table 3.
"Safe discharge" criteria.

9. Challenges and future

Considering the complexity and cost associated with hospital admissions and inpatient treatment, continuous shift in care from inpatient admission and treatment to outpatient care in the form of day care surgery has been witnessed globally in recent years [13]. Office procedure, OPD care and minor surgery were first included in day care surgery but with advancement of skill, technology and infrastructure even major surgery with proper preoperative work up, modern anesthesia and proper post-operative care with communications properly, adequate transport and back up plans to manage the complications with round the clock operation theater team with anesthesia team in alert and prepared mode for the any events to be managed in the operation theater. Development of health sector in new dimensions with development of day care surgery is optimum utilization of the resources and conserving the scarce fund of the patient for the payment of hospital bills very true and innovation for the underdeveloped nations. On the other hand, in developed nations, day care surgery almost crossed the half mark of all elective surgeries many years back and now almost 75% of the all elective surgeries are day care surgery. The challenges associated with establishment of day care surgery services are many and may appear at first review, insurmountable and may include lack of guidelines, lack of regulatory bodies and lack of supervision in poorly developed parts of the globes. Standard protocols and practices may be defined and set to identify the core concept of day care surgery. First challenge is upgradation of present health services to gear up for practice and all-elective acceptance of the day care surgery. Although there are still problems to be solved at the national level, such as training, this should not hinder the exploration of the development of local services. This is not necessarily very complicated. Simple methods such as the plan, execute, research and act (PDSA) cycle can be a very effective tool for initiating change, because the roles and perspectives of all relevant clinical and management resource groups are determined from the beginning. The plan here is the service change to be implemented (for example, to start a level 2 community surgery service). This involves mapping patient paths to show all relevant procedures and administrative processes surrounding patient management, thereby identifying potential gaps, bottlenecks, and barriers to change. During this process, questions about meeting visit goals, advance appointments, labor, capital flow, facilities, multidisciplinary team agreements, and patient information adequacy can be identified. To do is to implement changes to the service, rather than introducing this "wholesaler", it is better to test a small number of patients first to assess the impact. Research involves collecting data before and after implementing changes to observe and learn from the consequences. The bill involves determining what changes need to be made before it is fully implemented. Community surgical pathway planning should not be based on cost reduction, because experience shows that if community capacity meets previously unrecognized but clinically relevant needs, the costs of services may increase.

Second and biggest challenge is scope of day care surgery expansion which is limited by poor resource, technology limitations and infrastructure development and many advanced endoscopic, laparoscopic and intervention radiology procedures may not be included in day care surgery due to above limitations. Endocrine surgery, laparoscopic hernioplasty, laparoscopic cholecystectomy and laparoscopic fundoplication may be always in day care surgery with technology, skill and infrastructure. Proper post-operative care after use of an updated and advanced modern anesthesia system is essential in all day care surgery for acceptance in practice as well as patient centric outcomes [14, 15].

10. Summary

In summary, delivery of more surgery in primary care has potential for enhancing patient-centered management by promoting the development of multi-specialty community providers and reducing length of hospital stay. Finally, the outpatient surgical centers provide many benefits and advantages for surgical patients with proper organizations, dedicated services, and meticulous procedures.

Author details

Satyendra K. Tiwary
Department of General Surgery, Institute of Medical Sciences, Banaras Hindu University, Varanasi, India

*Address all correspondence to: satyendrak.tiwary1@bhu.ac.in

References

[1] Jarrett PEM, Roberts LM. Planning and designing a Day Surgery Unit. In: Lemos P, Jarrett P, Philip B, editors. Day Surgery Development and Practice. London, UK: International Association for Ambulatory Surgery (IAAS); 2006. pp. 61-87.

[2] Ruckley CV. Day care and short stay surgery for hernia. Br J Surg 1978; 65:1-4.

[3] Bailey CR, Ahuja M, Bartholomew K, Bew S, Forbes L, Lipp A, Montgomery J, Russon K, Potparic O, Stocker M. Guidelines for day-case surgery 2019: Guidelines from the Association of Anaesthetists and the British Association of Day Surgery. Anaesthesia. 2019 Jun;74(6):778-792. doi: 10.1111/anae.14639. Epub 2019 Apr 8. PMID: 30963557.

[4] Ansell GL, Montgomery JE. Outcome of ASA III patients undergoing day case surgery. Br J Anaesth. 2004 Jan;92(1): 71-74. doi: 10.1093/bja/aeh012. PMID: 14665556.

[5] Walsh MT. Improving outcomes in ambulatory anesthesia by identifying high risk patients. Curr Opin Anaesthesiol. 2018 Dec;31(6):659-666. doi: 10.1097/ACO.0000000000000653. PMID: 30325340.

[6] Atkins M, White J, Ahmed K. Day surgery and body mass index: results of a national survey. Anaesthesia. 2002 Feb;57(2):180-182. doi: 10.1046/j. 0003-2409.2001.02395.x. PMID: 11871956.

[7] Hao XY, Shen YF, Wei YG, Liu F, Li HY, Li B. Safety and effectiveness of day-surgery laparoscopic cholecystectomy is still uncertain: meta-analysis of eight randomized controlled trials based on GRADE approach. Surg Endosc. 2017 Dec;31(12):4950-4963. doi: 10.1007/ s00464-017-5610-1. Epub 2017 Jun 7. PMID: 28593414.

[8] Harsoor S. Changing concepts in anaesthesia for day care surgery. Indian J Anaesth. 2010 Nov;54(6):485-8. doi: 10.4103/0019-5049.72635. PMID: 21224963; PMCID: PMC3016566.

[9] Gangadhar S, Gopal T, Sathyabhama, Paramesh K. Rapid emergence of day-care anaesthesia: A review. Indian J Anaesth. 2012 Jul;56(4):336-41. doi: 10.4103/0019-5049.100813. PMID: 23087454; PMCID: PMC3469910.

[10] Association of Anaesthetists of Great Britain and Ireland; British Association of Day Surgery. Day case and short stay surgery: 2. Anaesthesia. 2011 May;66(5):417-434. doi: 10.1111/j.1365-2044.2011.06651.x. Epub 2011 Mar 18. PMID: 21418041.

[11] Bajwa SS, Bajwa SK, Kaur J, Sharma V, Singh A, Singh A, Goraya S, Parmar S, Singh K. Palonosetron: A novel approach to control postoperative nausea and vomiting in day care surgery. Saudi J Anaesth. 2011 Jan;5(1):19-24. doi: 10.4103/1658-354X.76484. PMID: 21655011; PMCID: PMC3101747.

[12] Ljungqvist O, Scott M, Fearon KC. Enhanced Recovery After Surgery: A Review. JAMA Surg. 2017 Mar 1;152(3):292-298. doi: 10.1001/ jamasurg.2016.4952. PMID: 28097305.

[13] Stessel B, Fiddelers AA, Joosten EA, Hoofwijk DMN, Gramke HF, Buhre WFFA. Prevalence and Predictors of Quality of Recovery at Home After Day Surgery. Medicine (Baltimore). 2015 Sep;94(39):e1553. doi: 10.1097/ MD.0000000000001553. PMID: 26426622; PMCID: PMC4616829.

[14] Fortier J, Chung F, Su J. Unanticipated admission after ambulatory surgery--a prospective

study. Can J Anaesth. 1998 Jul;45(7):612-619. doi: 10.1007/BF03012088. PMID: 9717590.

[15] Awad IT, Chung F. Factors affecting recovery and discharge following ambulatory surgery. Can J Anaesth 2006;53:858-872.

Chapter 9

Ambulatory Surgery for Perianal Disease

Andrea Divizia and Giuseppe S. Sica

Abstract

The gold standard in the diagnosis and treatment of proctological diseases is the exploration of the anal canal and distal rectum under anaesthesia (EUA), routinely performed as day case surgery. In selected cases it can be conducted as an outpatient exploration (OE) during a specialist surgical consultation. In the outpatient setting it is possible and safe to perform rubber band ligation, sclerotherapy and infrared coagulation for the treatment of haemorrhoidal disease, excision and incision of thrombosed external haemorrhoids, abscess drainage, setonage and fistulotomy also in case of perianal Crohn's disease, anal warts and skin tags removal. In terms of patients' satisfaction and success rate OE is comparable to EUA. All procedures can be performed under local anaesthesia. Pain control after the procedure is provided by oral pain killers.

Keywords: outpatients exploration, haemorrhoids, abscess and anal fistula, skin tags, anal warts, perianal Crohn's disease

1. Introduction

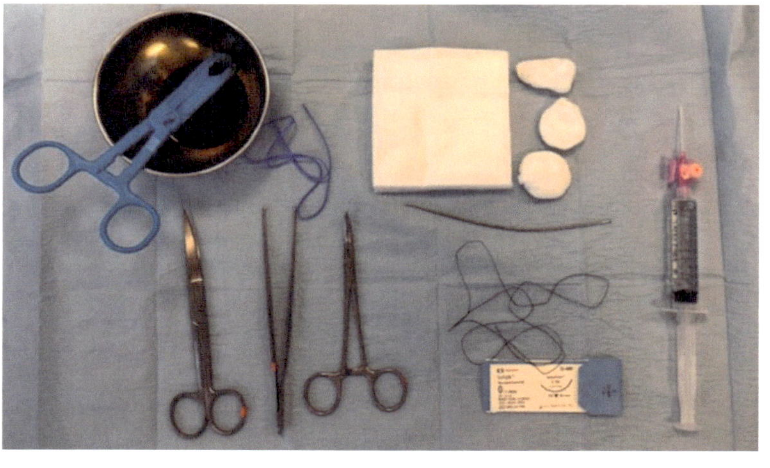

In the last decades, efforts and resources have been focused on developing health care services, resulting in newer facilities, greater resources of equipment and improved staffing, so that nowadays, surgical procedures can be carried out in large hospitals, providing both surgeons and patients safety and comfort. Consequently, not only major surgical interventions, but also minor procedures not requiring preoperative preparation, special equipment, nor hospital stay, are performed in these hospitals, thus tremendously increasing both the costs of medical treatment and the length of waiting lists for hospitalisation [1].

Recently, attention has shifted to outpatient care aiming to ensure safe surgical and medical assistance at reduced costs, spared resources and in shorter waiting times, through both office-based procedures, which include minor operation performed under local anaesthesia, requiring a short time to discharge (ranging from minutes to hours after the procedure) and day-surgery interventions, encompassing surgical operations more complex than office-based procedures, but easier than major surgery requiring at least an overnight stay [1, 2].

During the last 30 years, government with the support of health insurance companies, medical groups and hospital associations focused their concerted efforts on the development of proctologic office-based procedures in order to reduce hospital costs and release beds for major surgeries. While almost 30–50% of all surgeries can be safely realised in outpatient sectors, this rate raises to 90% in anorectal operations [1]. In fact, even if complications rate following anorectal office-based procedures are extremely variable, the majority of them are minor complications and do not require hospitalisation, nor further surgical intervention.

Factors appealing to physicians include significant costs saving achieved avoiding the cost of admission, use of ward-based supplies, respiratory therapy, increased medication costs, and laboratory charges. Other advantages include lack of need to perform trichotomy, prophylactic antibiotic treatment, and enema administration. Moreover, also patients' satisfaction degree is increased thanks to the ease of scheduling cases, the advantage of avoiding a hospital stay and the early return home [1, 3].

However, to perform ambulatory anorectal surgery, a proper patient selection is necessary. Patient comorbidities as well as functional limitations should be assessed. The type and extent of surgery should be considered since not all anorectal procedures are minor [3].

2. Patient position

Patient positioning during proctologic assessment is important for patients and doctors. Patients undergoing both proctologic examination and ambulatory procedures are usually embarrassed because they lay naked on uncomfortable position, that can be:

- Sims' position, or left lateral position
- Lithotomy position with lifted legs, or gynaecological position
- Knee–chest position
- Knee–chest position with patients body bent forward, or jack-knife position

Even though the majority of individuals would favour Sims' position if they had the choice, they do not feel less embarrassed, thus preferring to let doctors free to choose the most suitable position to get reliable diagnoses of anal complaints [4]. The most performed positions are left lateral Sims' position and jack-knife position. The former is more comfortable for the patients and is easily and quickly achieved by the patient itself, allowing doctors to save time. This position is the most suitable to analyse haemorrhoids, but can be adapted to each proctologic disease. The jack-knife position, on the contrary, requires a scissoring table able to lift the hip, letting head and legs down and takes more time to be obtained. The sloping position of the patient makes it difficult to analyse haemorrhoids, however as the buttocks fall to each side, and finger tips of both hands of the investigator are free, it provides a better field of view on anal and perianal surface in good lighting. Since sensitivity, specificity, and the predictive value of anal diagnoses in different proctological positions are unknown, and considering that none of different proctological positionings are most embarrassing to patients, doctors choice usually depends on their own customs and preferences.

3. Anaesthesia

Ambulatory anaesthesia has to provide a rapid onset analgesic effect, ensuring pain control and allowing an early discharge after the treatment is performed. The choice of the intra-operative anaesthetic management should consider patient's related factors, such as age, clinical condition and preference, surgeons' preference and procedural related factors, such as the kind of treatment and its length [5]. Anaesthesia for ambulatory procedures ranges from local to loco-regional anaesthesia, including pudendal nerve block and posterior perineal block; however, the easiest and shortest therapeutic sessions could even be performed without any anaesthesia, paying attention to the post-operative management, especially in terms of post-operative pain control.

Local anaesthesia is obtained through subcutaneous, intradermal or submucosal 1% lidocaine injections. Complications rate following local anaesthesia are extremely low, thus allowing to safely perform it in an outpatient setting. They include pain, which is usually due to the injected anaesthetic volume causing tissue distension, allergic reactions, and infections. Cardiovascular collapse is a rare but potentially life-threatening complication, requiring promptly intubation and vosoactive substances, steroids and myorelaxant drugs administration. Local anaesthesia is a quick and easy to perform anaesthesia, that allows performing minor ambulatory procedures, keeping pain under control.

Loco-regional anaesthesia includes pudendal nerve block and posterior perineal block. Pudendal nerve block, firstly described by Mueller in 1908, is performed with the patient in gynaecological position and is usually preceded by local anaesthesia administration if carried out in an ambulatory setting to an awake patient. After identifying the ischial spine, the needle punctures the skin transperineally, medial to the ischial tuberosity, 2–3 centimetres away from the anal margin. The needle is advanced in the posterolateral direction until the ischial spine and then rotated in the medial inferior direction to the ischial spine, passing through the sacrospinous ligament. After negative aspiration, the local anaesthetic, usually ropivacaina, is injected. Posterior perineal block, also known as Marti's technique, is performed with the patient in gynaecological or lithotomic position and preceded –in case of outpatient setting, by local anaesthesia administration, just as for pudendal nerve block. It involves infiltration of the inferior hemorrhoidal nerves, the posterior branch of the internal pudendal nerves, and the anococcygeal nerves and block of the inferior gluteal nerves and of perineal branches of minor nerves from the sacral plexus. It is achieved injecting ropivacaina or lidocaine 2 cm from the anal verge in the posterior commissure, 8 to 10 centimetres deeply into each ischiorectal fossa and superficially in the anterior commissure to achieve a complete infiltration of the perineal skin. Loco-regional anaesthesia is usually suitable to perform exploration under anaesthesia (EUA) of the anal canal in operative theatre and is associated to general anaesthesia to reach a complete multimodal pain control. In the ambulatory setting loco-regional techniques are unfrequently used, but sometimes may be required to perform more invasive treatments. Complications are the same as for local anaesthesia, thus even if more invasive than local anaesthesia, these techniques may be safely performed for outpatient treatment.

4. Postoperative management

Postoperative management after proctologic office-based procedures mostly focuses on post-procedural pain control. It starts with anaesthesia performed during the procedure, so that the dose of analgesic drugs thereafter required is reduced and recovery time and return to daily living activities are shortened. After office-based procedures the pain can be controlled with oral pain killers administration. While the use of non-steroidal anti-inflammatory drugs (NSAIDs) alone is poorly effective to control severe pain and the use of narcotics alone may cause various side effects such as nausea, vomiting, dizziness and constipation (thus ultimately exacerbating pain symptoms), multimodal or balanced analgesia is the most effective treatment. It consists of administering in addition to narcotics, drugs with different mechanisms of actions and target pathways, including NSAIDs, acetaminophen, gabapentinoids, dexamethasone, alpha 2 agonists, NMDA receptor antagonists, and duloxetine. Acetaminophen and NSAIDs such as ketorolac and ibunoprofen successfully manage pain, resulting in an effective narcotic-sparing approach. The administration of pain killers drugs belonging to different classes results in increased analgesic effect and reduced drugs-induced side effects [5–7].

Analgesia may be provided by lidocaine and prilocaine ointment, too, ensuring supplemental pain relief and furtherly sparing narcotics.

Besides oral pain killers administration and local analgesic ointments application, anal burning and patient satisfaction may be improved by warn sitz baths. They are considered a worthwhile potential adjunct with little associated risk even if do not significantly reduce actual pain. Sitz baths or showers starting within 24 hours of the operation should be performed three times per day and after bowel movements for comfort and cleanliness [8].

Finally, to ensure pain control, it is fundamental to avoid constipation. Usually increased dietary fibre and fluid intake is sufficient to reduce postoperative constipation and pain upon defecation. However, even if dietary modification could guarantee stool softening, some physicians feel more comfortable recommending stimulant laxatives and stool softeners [5].

Postoperative management includes also follow-up instructions and written discharge instructions, improving patient satisfaction and decreasing the need for patients to seek additional medical attention, thus even reducing costs.

5. Haemorrhoids

Haemorrhoids are arteriovenous sinusoids, located in the sub-epithelial space, embedded in connective tissue and smooth muscle fibres, participating to 15–20% of the anal continence [9–12]. Haemorrhoidal disease (HD) is characterised by abnormally congested and downward displaced haemorrhoids [11–13].

HD is one of the most frequent medical and surgical diseases and the commonest proctologic disease, experienced by more than 50% of the population over 50 years old in various degree. Reports on HD prevalence rate widely varies (4,4–39%) [9, 14–16] because clinical manifestations may overlap with those of others anorectal diseases and may be wrongly attributed to other proctologic conditions; moreover many patients are asymptomatic, not requiring any treatment, while others self-diagnose and self-manage without referring to a specialist.

Increased intraabdominal pressure due to constipation and prolonged straining are the commonest conditions leading to haemorrhoidal disease because of obstruction of venous return, resulting in engorgement of the haemorrhoidal plexus [17]. Moreover, defecation of hard faecal material increases shearing force on the anal cushions.

Painless rectal bleeding is the commonest onset of haemorrhoidal disease, which may present as minimal bright red bleeding per rectum or hematochezia after bowel movements [18–20], or even severe acute lower gastrointestinal bleeding requiring hospitalisation and blood transfusion in the most severe cases [17, 19]. Although rectal bleeding is the commonest sign of HD, less frequent presentations may be prolapse (even determining difficult defecation), mucous discharge, swelling, soiling, perianal skin irritation, itching, feeling of a lump, and discomfort. Acute anal pain is rarely a presentation symptoms, appearing only in case of thrombosed external haemorrhoids.

Despite such a variable clinical onset, HD diagnosis is easily achieved collecting the medical history and performing a physical examination including abdominal examination, and a local examination with the patient on a left lateral position, including inspection of the perianal tissues, anorectal digital examination, and anoscopy. However, even if haemorrhoids are easily recognised, it is necessary to perform an endoscopic examination to exclude more severe colorectal conditions [17].

Once HD has been diagnosed, the chosen treatment depends on haemorrhoids location, on the severity of the disease and on an eventual previously administered treatment. Haemorrhoids location refers to the dentate line, allowing a distinction between internal (above the dentate line and covered with mucosa) and external haemorrhoids (below the dentate line and coated with squamous epithelium), which differ not only for their position, but also blood supply, drainage, epithelization and innervations [20]. In particular, internal haemorrhoids receive visceral innervations and are less sensitive to pain, thus amenable to office-based treatment performed without or with minimal anaesthesia. On the contrary, external haemorrhoids are more sensitive to pain receiving somatic innervations and, therefore, require surgical treatment performed under anaesthesia, thrombosed external haemorrhoids being the only exception.

Regarding to haemorrhoids severity, while no widely accepted classification exists for external haemorrhoids, the extent of internal haemorrhoids is usually assessed with the Goligher classification [10, 17, 21], depending on the degree to which they prolapse from the anal canal, so that bleeding without prolapse stands for grade I, haemorrhoidal piles prolapsing during straining correspond to grade II and III if they respectively reduce spontaneously or manually, and non reducible haemorrhoids are classified as grade IV. As the grade becomes worse, office-based procedures or surgery are required. In particular grade I treatment is usually conservative, grade II and III are amenable of office-based procedures, and grade IV haemorrhoids require surgery.

However, even if the chosen treatment depends on both haemorrhoids location and severity degree, usually the first therapeutic step is conservative and consists on dietary and lifestyle modifications, if necessary associated to topical or oral medication. Conservative treatment is successful for the majority of patients and could be periodically administered for as long as the patient wishes. If conservative treatment fails or the patient chooses a more invasive approach, office-based procedures or surgery are indicated [12, 14, 22].

5.1 Outpatient treatment

Outpatient treatment is recommended for symptomatic patients affected by grade I, II or III haemorrhoidal disease refractory to conservative treatment [12, 14, 22]. It encompasses rubber band ligation, sclerotherapy, infrared coagulation, excision of thrombosed external haemorrhoids and few other techniques, not frequently used, such as electrotherapy, HET bipolar system, YAG or carbon dioxide laser and cryo-surgery [23]. Their common aim is to slough haemorrhoidal tissue and generate a scar so that residual tissue is fixated to the underlying sub-mucosal tissue and anorectal muscular ring. Each procedure is adopted in specific circumstances, being rubber band ligation the most frequently performed with a wider therapeutic range. Even if they differ for technical features and indications, all the office-based procedures are characterised by faster recovery and less pain than surgical treatment [24]. Moreover, complication rate following outpatient treatment is extremely low, varying between post-procedural pain –usually easy-controlled by oral painkillers, to perineal sepsis –the most severe and life threatening condition, which is extremely rare.

Ambulatory procedures may require more than one treatment session and can be repeated until a complete response, if the patient agrees. In fact, since haemorrhoidal disease is not a severe clinical condition, it is up to the patient whether to manage them with a conservative approach or surgery. Choice of the outpatient treatment should take into consideration patient preferences, availability of procedures and fitness for further procedures. Only in case of coexisting internal haemorrhoids and additional anorectal pathologies surgery should be suggested as first line treatment [12, 14, 22].

5.2 Rubber band ligation

Rubber band ligation (RBL) is the most commonly performed office-based treatment, having the widest therapeutic range and the highest success rate. This procedure is recommended to treat almost all patients affected by symptomatic internal haemorrhoids refractory to conservative treatment, being contraindicated only in few cases:

- Grade IV internal haemorrhoids, since symptoms improvement is registered in less than 50% of cases

- Thrombosed haemorrhoids, characterised by excruciating pain that makes the procedure impossible to be performed

- Anticoagulant therapy or coagulation disorders, because of the increased risk of delayed haemorrhage [25]

- Immunodeficiency and diabetes mellitus, because of the increased risk of infection and sepsis [26]

- Concomitant anorectal diseases, for which surgery should be the first line treatment

- Pregnancy, usually determining a transient condition, requiring a conservative treatment

During the procedure, patients lay on left lateral position or semi-inverted jack-knife position, being the former more comfortable for the patient. The anoscope is essential to perform the procedure, consisting on the positioning of a rubber band on the base of the haemorrhoid, at least 5 mm above the dentate line. The application of the elastic band causes immediate ischemic damage and 3 to 5 days delayed necrosis, leading to a localised sub-mucosal scarring that secures the mucosal layers to the underlying tissues. Rubber band application may be performed using both forceps or suction devices [27, 28]. The former represents the traditional technique but requires two people to be performed: the operator and the assistance, whose role is to hold the anoscope. The latter includes both endoscopic suction devices and vacuum suction devices, which allow the operator to hold both the ligator and the anoscope, performing the procedure without any assistant.

Usually just one pile per session is treated, in order to reduce procedure-related risks. Multiple sessions should be performed in 4-week intervals, to allow a complete recovery from the previous treatment [29].

If the procedure is correctly performed, with the rubber band placed at least 5 mm above the dentate line, the patient has no pain, thus the procedure can safely be performed without any anaesthesia. Whenever the patient experiences pain, the band is wrongly placed below the dentate line, onto somatically innervated tissue, and should promptly be removed. Beside pain, that occurs in almost 8% of the procedures and is most frequently due to band misplacement [30], other extremely rare complications include [31–34]:

- Bleeding
- Thrombosis
- Skin tags
- Localised infection
- Liver abscesses
- Endocarditis
- Perineal sepsis
- Death

RBL is the most effective office-based procedures, improving symptoms in 93–100% of patients having grade II haemorrhoids and 78–84% of those having grade III haemorrhoids and reducing bleeding in up to 90% of patients [30, 35]. When compared to haemorrhoid artery ligation (HAL), it shows lower rates of bleeding, intra- and post-procedural pain, but higher risk of recurrences. The same has to be said comparing RBL to surgery: the former has a reduced complication risk compared to surgery, while the latter has lower recurrence rates [36].

5.3 Sclerotherapy

Sclerotherapy is the second most frequently performed outpatient procedure for haemorrhoidal disease. Since bleeding and infection risk is lower than after rubber band ligation, this procedure finds application whenever RBL cannot be performed, thus it is recommended for patients on anticoagulant therapy or coagulation disorders and in case of immunodeficiency or other pathological conditions increasing infective risks [35].

As for RBL, the procedure is performed through an anoscope, with the patient laying on left lateral position. Sclerosing solutions are injected into the submucosa plane above the dentate line, so that the treatment does not require any anaesthesia, and determine an intense inflammatory reaction that leads to scarring and adhesion of haemorrhoids to the underlying tissue just like after ligation with elastic bands.

The most frequently used solutions are aluminium potassium sulphate and tannic acid (ALTA, which seems to be the most effective) [37–39], 5% phenol in vegetable oil and 50% dextrose water.

Complications following sclerotherapy are even rarer than after RBL, considering patients major complain is painful intra-procedural injection, reported in almost 90% of cases, while post-procedural pain is experienced only by 25–50% of patients. Bleeding is uncommon and in the majority of cases is a self-limited condition following injection. The most frequent post-operative complication is mucosal necrosis, which is reported in less than 4% of patients and is usually caused by too superficial injections (not reaching the submucosal layer). Rare but major complications include impotence, fatal necrotising fasciitis, rectourethral fistulas, and rectal perforations, that are mostly ascribed to misplaced injections –both in non haemorrhoidal tissue or in the vascular system [40].

Sclerotherapy successfully manage haemorrhoidal bleeding, leading to an improvement in 100% of patients with second and third degree haemorrhoids [35, 39]. Moreover it leads to a complete resolution of symptoms in 88% of I degree haemorrhoids and 52% III degree haemorrhoids. However, even if much safer than RBL and despite its high success rate, recurrences are more frequent in patients undergoing sclerotherapy than ligation with elastic bands, thus the latter resulting as the preferred choice for both surgeons and patients whenever not contraindicated [41].

5.4 Infrared coagulation

Infrared coagulation (IC) is an outpatient procedure indicated for the treatment of refractory to conservative treatment grade I, II and III haemorrhoidal disease [12, 14]. In literature, data regarding IC treatment are extremely variable, ranging from studies showing similar results as for sclerotherapy, to papers underlying higher recurrence rates with fewer post-procedural complications and less intra-procedural discomfort. Thus, whether to use infrared coagulation or sclerotherapy depends on availability of procedures and surgeon preferences.

Infrared coagulation is also performed through an anoscope, with the patient laying in the same position as for the previous procedures. It consists of infrared light waves application on the haemorrhoidal tissue above the dentate line, which are converted into heat determining an immediate protein coagulation and necrosis, visible as 3 mm wide and 3 mm deep white spot on the mucosa. The treatment of each haemorrhoid cushion may require from three to five applications. As for the other office-based procedures, IC causes a scar fixating the redundant haemorrhoidal mucosa to the underlying tissues.

Complications following infrared coagulation include pain, which is the most frequent occurring in 16–100% of patients and bleeding, which ranges from 15 to 45% of cases [42, 43]. Moreover, many studies report high frequency of persistency and recurrence after the treatment: recurrence rate is estimated to be about 15% at three months.

Success rates reported by a recent meta-analysis widely range from 22 to 51 and 78%, when considering respectively grade III, II and I haemorrhoidal disease [35, 43].

5.5 Excision and incision of thrombosed external haemorrhoids

Haemorrhoidal excision is a procedure that can be performed both in an office-based setting and in the operating theatre. It is the only office-based procedure suitable for the treatment of external haemorrhoids, which are localised below the dentate line, have somatic innervation and thus are more sensitive to pain, making surgery performed in the operating theatre the best therapeutic option.

Thrombosed external haemorrhoids belong to the so called anorectal emergencies. They occur with an acutely painful purplish or blue mass in the perianal area that gradually reduces after the first couple of days; bleeding may present in case the high pressure within the thrombus causes overlying skin erosion. It is important to differentiate this pathologic condition from complicated internal haemorrhoids and anal pigmented melanoma, whose onset in similar being characterised by perianal pain. External haemorrhoids are covered with anoderm and usually suddenly appear, while internal haemorrhoids are covered with mucosa and anal pigmented melanoma has a long story of pigmented skin lesion [44].

Excision of the thrombosed external haemorrhoids is indicated for patients experiencing persistent pain from 72 hours or less, providing immediate relief [45]. After 48 to 72 hours, the thrombus organises and contracts, diminishing symptoms so that a conservative management can be proposed, obviating the need for surgical management. Surgical treatment for thrombosed external haemorrhoids may be required also in case of residual skin tags resulting from the healing process of a small ulcer following a spontaneous evacuation of a thrombosed haemorrhoid. However, residual skin tags rarely cause enough symptoms to warrant its removal; only in case of large skin tags determining skin irritation, itching, pain, or inability to keep proper hygiene, excision can be beneficial.

The office-based procedure to treat thrombosed external haemorrhoids include excision and incision. The former can be performed in the operating room as well as in an appropriately equipped office. After the administration of both local anaesthesia and anal block, the excision of a thrombosed haemorrhoid is performed by making an elliptical incision in the overlying skin. A careful dissection of the haemorrhoid from the superficial fibres of the anal sphincter is carried out, trying to avoid injury. Thereafter skin edges can be left open allowing drainage or reapproximated with absorbable sutures [46]. Topical antibiotic ointments are not routinely applied as infections are rare in this well-vascularized sites.

Inexperienced physicians, unable to perform haemorrhoids excision, can manage this anorectal emergency with a simple incision of the overlying skin, allowing evacuation of thrombus, thus producing immediate relief of pain.

However, incision and evacuation of the clot is associated with a 30% risk of reaccumulation and thrombosis, which may disseminate to adjacent hemorrhoidal columns [47], thus this technique is not recommended and whenever performed requires a follow-up within the next 24 to 48 hours for surgical evaluation. On the contrary, recurrence rate for a completely excised thrombosed hemorrhoid is lower (5–19%) [48, 49].

If surgery is not feasible, conservative management would be offered including anti-inflammatory analgesics, warm sitz bath, reducing activity and avoiding constipation. Education and reassurance about this condition and its benign nature would be beneficial to the patient.

6. Abscess and anal fistula

Abscesses and anal fistulas are common anorectal problems, representing two different phases of the same infectious process. Perianal and perirectal abscesses are acute infections, resulting in pus collection, mostly due to non-specific cryptoglandular obstruction [50]. Anorectal fistulas represent the chronic evolution of a suppurative process, characterised by an epithelised tract connecting two epithelised surfaces, in particular anal or rectal mucosa to the perianal skin or perineum [51, 52].

Estimated anal abscess incidence is about 2 cases per 10,000 population per year [53, 54], leading to fistula formation in about 25% of patients. Fistulas may present de novo, but in about 30–50% of patients, they follow a previous anorectal abscess. Both anal abscesses and fistulas affect men twice more than women, having a mean age of presentation of 40 years (ranging from 20 to 60 years). However, since most patients attribute proctologic symptoms to haemorrhoidal disease without referring to a specialist, abscesses and fistulas real incidence is unknown.

As previously said, both anal abscesses and fistulas usually originate from obstructed anal crypt glands. Less frequently they can be caused by inflammatory bowel disease (mainly Crohn's disease), infection such as actinomycosis, tuberculosis and lymphogranuloma venereum, human immunodeficiency virus, trauma (both in case of iatrogenic injuries and foreign rectal bodies), surgery, malignancy and irradiation [50, 55].

The commonest onset of a perianal abscess is constant severe pain, usually not related to bowel movements, that can be associated to general symptoms such as fever or generalised malaise [52]. On the contrary, intermittent perianal pain exacerbated by bowel movements and chronic purulent drainage are typical manifestations of fistulas [56].

On physical examination, abscesses present as erythematous, tender and fluctuant masses; purulent drainage, either from the overlying skin or from the rectum, can be present if the abscess has begun to spontaneously drain [52]. On the contrary, the presence of an external opening draining pus and a palpable cord leading from the detected external orifice to an internal orifice, are the most common findings in case of anal fistula [56].

Although collecting the medical history and performing a physical examination allow to detect the majority of abscesses and fistulas, sometimes patients may not have any physical finding on examination, and further instrumental exams may be required. Local examination may result difficult in case of deep abscesses, not appreciable on external examination nor by digitorectal examination, and in case of incomplete or blind-ended fistulas, lacking of the external orifice. Moreover, symptoms of both conditions may overlap with the clinical manifestations of other proctologic diseases. In these cases and in case of complex or recurrent fistulas, imaging is necessary [57, 58]. The most commonly performed imaging studies are magnetic resonance imaging (MRI), which is the gold standard imaging technique, and endosonography (EUS), having a specificity of 69% and 43% respectively, and the same sensitivity of 87% [58–60]. Instrumental investigation gives important information about abscess localisation, fistula anatomy and integrity of the sphincter muscles, allowing to establish the proper treatment.

In case of anal abscesses, the required treatment is always a prompt drainage, considering that all undrained abscess can expand toward adjacent spaces or progress to a systemic infection [56, 57]. Surgical approach may vary depending on imaging findings, that allow to classify an abscess as follow:

- Simple anorectal abscess, or perianal abscess
- Complex anorectal abscess, including:

- ○ Ischiorectal abscess, which extended through the external anal sphincter into the ischiorectal space

- ○ Intersphincteric abscess, located in the intersphincteric groove

- ○ Supraelevator abscess, reaching the supralevator space and originating from cryptoglandular infection or pelvic inflammatory processes

- ○ Horseshoe abscess, rising posteriorly to the anal canal and extending to the ischiorectal space

According to this classification, perianal abscesses treatment can be safely performed in an outpatient setting, while in case of complex, large or deep abscesses, drainage should be performed in the operating room, under general anaesthesia, sedation or local anaesthesia [61].

Anorectal fistula management is quite more difficult, considering the chosen surgical treatment depends on the relation between the fistula tract and the external anal sphincter, and on the amount of the sphincter complex involved with the fistulous tract. According to Parks' classification, firstly described in 1976, four different types of anal fistula can be identified based on the relationship between the primary track and the sphincter [62]:

- Parks type 1, intersphincteric fistula (45%), which extend between internal and external sphincter

- Parks type 2, transsphinteric fistula (30%), passing through internal and external sphincter, reaching perineum

- Parks type 3, sovrasphincteric fistula (20%), which encircles both internal and external sphincters, reaching the ischiorectal fossa

- Parks type 4, extrasphincteric fistula (3%), which encompasses the entire sphincter apparatus, including the levators, reaching the skin overlying the buttock; this fistula usually does not come from a cryptoglandular abscess

- Superficial, not involving any sphincter muscle (not included in the original Parks classification)

A fistula can also be categorised as simple or complex. The former includes those with an intersphincteric or low transsphincteric track that involves less than 30% of the sphincter complex. A fistula in the presence of inflammatory bowel disease, malignancy, incontinence, chronic diarrhoea or previous irradiation should be considered complex as well as those with an anterior track in a female patient [63]. In some complex cases, a staged surgical procedure will be required.

Since perianal infection sequelae range from minor pain and social embarrassment due to smelly purulent drainage, to life-threatening sepsis, once a diagnosis is established, surgery is the mainstay of the treatment, aiming to resolve local infection, remove fistulous tracts, avoid recurrences and preserve sphincteric function.

6.1 Abscess drainage

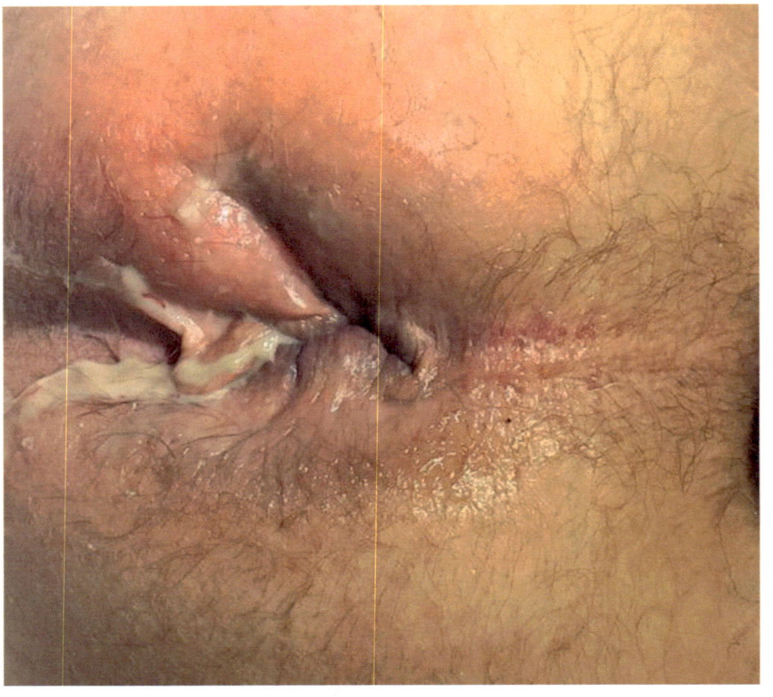

Abscess incision and drainage is a procedure that can be performed either under local anaesthesia, in an ambulatory setting, whenever the pus collection is small and superficial, either under general anaesthesia, sedation or local anaesthesia in the operating room, in case of more complex, larger or deeper abscesses [56, 57]. In these cases an office-based treatment can be performed only in referral centres if carried out by expert surgeons.

Incision should be performed as close as possible to the anal verge minimising the length of a potential fistula while still providing adequate drainage of the collection. As 30–70% of abscesses present with a concomitant fistula, surgeons question whether to perform or not a primary fistulotomy with the abscess drainage [64–67]. Data regarding this argument show primary fistulotomy reduces the risk of recurrence and persistence of the disease, but increase sphincter damage risk even leading to faecal incontinence [56, 57, 68]. Thus, primary fistulotomy is recommended only in case of simple anal fistula or high recurrence risk.

While perianal abscesses (simple abscesses) may be treated in an ambulatory setting, complex abscesses usually require an operating theatre, except for small intersphincteric abscesses, that can be managed without requiring an exploration under anaesthesia (EUA).

Regardless of the surgical setting, a course of empiric antibiotics is strongly recommended for all patients who went through incision and drainage of an anorectal abscess, in order to reduce the rate of fistula formation. Recommended drugs are amoxicillin-clavulanate or a combination of ciprofloxacin and metronidazole, administered for a four- to five-day course [69]. However, even if this treatment reduces fistula recurrence rate, it does not affect abscess recurrence rate [70].

6.2 Setonage and fistulotomy

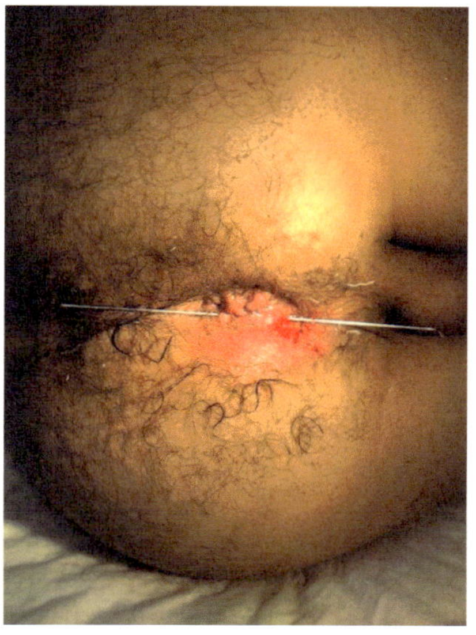

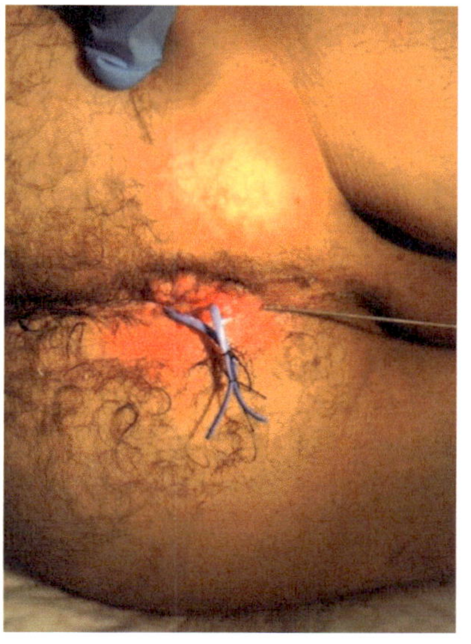

Setonage and fistulotomy represent the gold standard for the treatment of anorectal fistulas and can be performed both in an outpatient setting and in an operating room, depending on fistula anatomical features. The placement of a seton can be considered when the internal opening is identifiable. Fistulotomy can be carried out with a simultaneous drainage of the abscess in case of a simple fistula, or can be performed as a second stage procedure 4–8 weeks after drainage [56, 57].

Fistulotomy is performed with the patient laying on a left lateral position. After a probe is inserted into the external opening and gently passed along the fistula tract to the internal opening, an incision is made over the entire length of the fistula using the probe as a guide. The tract is then gently curetted and is left opened to heal for second-intention healing or marsupialised to promote healing, depending on surgeons preference. The most critical step in this procedure is to identify and curette the internal opening to reduce the risk of recurrence, since concomitant induration due to inflammation may obscure the internal opening. Hydrogen peroxide injected through the external orifice may help to identify the internal opening [66], while overzealous attempts with a fistula probe should be discouraged as they can cause iatrogenic damage [71].

The most concerning potential complication of a fistulotomy is incontinence (either to solid faeces or liquid faeces or gas) from procedure-related damageto the external anal sphincter. The reported rates of incontinence are highly variable, ranging from 0 to 82% [72, 73], with an increased risk if the fistulotomy is performed at the time of the drainage of an acute abscess [74]. Nevertheless, when fistulotomy is used forsimple anal fistulas in properly selected patients, the risk of faecal incontinence is minimal or none [75, 76].

This treatment is indicated to manage simple fistulas, thus superficial fistulas, intersphincteric fistulas and low transsphincteric fistulas, involving less than 30% of the sphincter complex. For these fistula it is an effective treatment with a high success rate ranging from 79 to 100% [77–79] and low recurrence rates [66, 72, 80, 81].

In females and in patients with preoperative impairment of continence, a high or recurrent fistula, previous fistula surgery or Crohn's disease, any division of the sphincter should be undertaken with caution and by an experienced surgeon [82]. The location of the internal opening per se, whether high or low in the anal canal, should not be used as a guide to "safe fistulotomy".

As fistulotomy, also the insertion of a seton through the fistula track is performed with the patient laying on a left lateral position and requires fistula track probing. Once the seton lays through the fistula track it can be used in different ways. A loose seton purpose is to facilitate drainage preventing an acute exacerbation of abscess formation and to allow healing of any secondary tracts, allowing local assessment some weeks later [57, 83]. A cutting seton purpose is to allow a gradual division of the sphincter, thank to a progressive tightening [57, 84]. Recently reported data of patients undergoing fistulotomy with a cutting seton tightened every 6–8 weeks, reported healing rates over 90% with only minor disturbances in anal sphincter function in 4% of patients [85–87].

Complex fistula treatment, including ligation of intersphincteric fistula tract (LIFT) [88, 89], advancement flap [90, 91], diversion, proctectomy and modified Haley procedure, cannot be performed in an office-based setting.

7. Perianal Crohn's disease

Crohn's disease (CD) is an idiopathic, incurable chronic inflammatory disease of the GI tract [92–95], associated in more than 30% of cases to symptoms of perianal disease (PAD) [96–98]. The risk of developing PAD is consistent with the time from the diagnosis of CD, from 20% after ten years and up to 30% after twenty years. However, PAD is far more common in patients with colon (41%) and rectum (90%) localization and less in patients with ileal disease (12%) [99–102]. Early diagnosis and correct treatment are crucial to allow patients to promptly start medical treatments with antitumor necrosis factor (tnf) which is considered the cornerstone of treatment, offering the best long-term control of PAD [103–116].

The gold standard to assess symptomatic perianal disease (PAD) in CD patients is the exploration of the anal canal and distal rectum under anaesthesia (EUA) [117–122]. EUA usually allows a correct diagnosis of fistulous tracts, a classification of the fistula, and an appropriate treatment of the PAD at the same time. In tertiary centres, PAD treatment can be performed also in an outpatient setting by expert surgeons. Whether to perform an EUA or an outpatient exploration (OE) depends on the anatomy, the type of fistula, and finally, the surgeon's expertise [123–129]. Moreover, active proctitis control must be achieved whenever possible prior to any surgical treatment. Treatment strategy and procedures are different in an acute or in an elective setting; in acute management, the main aim is sepsis control: incision and drainage of every abscess are strongly advised, while placement of a loose seton should be considered only if the fistulous tract can be promptly and easily identified [120]. In an elective setting, an exploration of the anal canal and distal rectum under anaesthesia is recommended and, in case of complex fistula, even in the presence of proctitis, a loose, draining seton could be passed if the internal and external orifices of the fistulous tract are found. A fistulotomy or fistulectomy can be safely considered for simple posterior fistulas [133].

Perianal fistulas in CD may be simple or complex according to the American Gastroenterological Association (AGA) [130–133]. Simple fistulas have a high healing rate, while complex fistulas are difficult to treat and show a poor healing rate and increased rate of relapse.

The aim of the surgical treatment of PAD in CD patients should be symptoms or complication control, allowing patients to pursue a timely medical therapy, in a multidisciplinary management. In the presence of a symptomatic perianal fistula, an optimal result can be considered to avoid sepsis, allowing for a good drainage before thinking to the complete healing of the fistula and finally preventing the recurrence and preserving the continence of the anal sphincter. It is essential to ensure timely treatment, because perianal fistulas significantly impair the quality of life of the patients, to avoid the potentially disastrous consequences such as those of an undrained sepsis or ramification of the fistulous tracts [134–139]. Only the patients with symptomatic Crohn's anal fistula should undergo a surgical treatment. The gold standard treatment for symptomatic perianal disease in CD patients is conducted during the EUA. Most of the series available in literature refer to day surgery or overnight admission. Unfortunately, a timely treatment is not always possible and this, as said, may well represent a relevant clinical issue.

According to the Association of Coloproctology of Great Britain and Ireland consensus conference on surgical management of fistulating perianal Crohn's disease, experienced surgeons should always try to place a seton when the fistulous tract is readily identifiable and this should be possible most of the times in "skilled hands". Compliance of patients to the procedure was high and, from a surgical point of view, the OE was nice to perform without difficulties or trouble in all cases.

This procedure should be offered in a high-volume center in which a multidisciplinary dedicated team is available. In selected cases, OE may be offered as a "bridge to surgery," able to faster solve critical clinical issues or palliate disabling symptoms with low morbidity and discomfort, also allowing patients to continue medical therapy. OE can be repeated, if necessary, in different occasion. From an economical point of view, the OE can definitively save logistics and money. The OE surely is a minimally invasive approach, with low morbidity and very low patient stress. OE could be a safe and effective procedure that can be proposed to the vast majority of patients with Crohn's fistulas. It is not recommended in nonexperienced hands and in high complex or rectovaginal fistulas (Hughes classification 1b, 1d or 2d, and 2e).

8. Anal warts

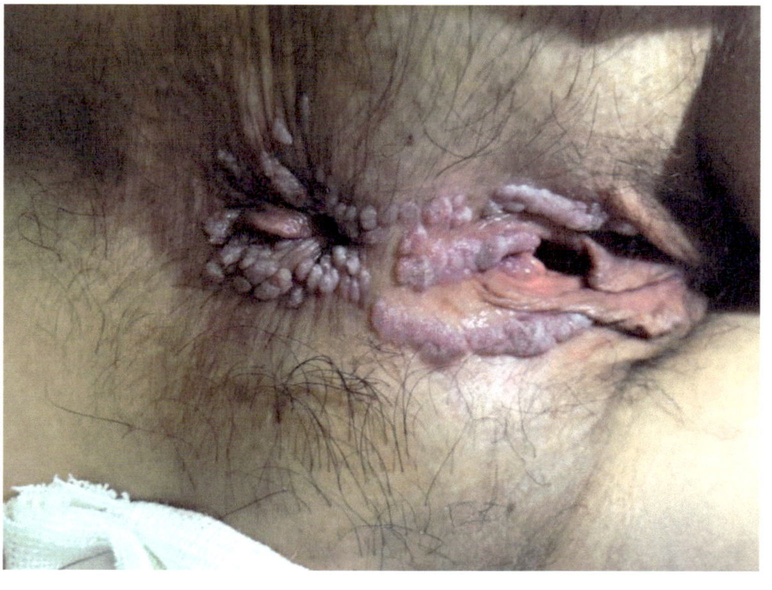

Anal warts, also known as condyloma acuminata, are growths of tissue localised in the area around and inside the anus, usually caused by human papillomavirus (HPV).

The Human Papilloma Virus (HPV) used to be thought as one of the most common sexually transmitted diseases (STds) [140]. The estimated incidence of HPV infection is high, with 14 million persons infected annually and 79 million persons with prevalent infection [141]. Its family (Papillomaviridae) consists of more than 120 viruses presenting a tropism toward either the cutaneous or mucosa epithelium, however the vast majority (90%) of anal warts are caused only by two low-risk HPV subtypes: 6 and 11 [142]. Further HPV-associated diseases include other mucocutaneous warts as well as cervical, anal, vaginal, vulvar, penile, and oropharyn-geal cancers.

Anogenital warts (AGWs) diagnosis is most often based on their clinical appearance, and tests for the presence of HPV are not recommended for their diagnosis. They firstly appear as tiny spots or growths, whose dimensions may rapidly increase even covering the anal area. Usually, they do not cause any pain or discomfort. Some patients may experience itching, bleeding, mucus discharge, or a feeling of a lump or mass in the area. Histologic examination of biopsy specimens can be performed to rule out intraepithelial or invasive squamous cell carcinomas (SCCs), which can coexist with or appear similar to AGWs.

Therapeutic options for the treatment of anal warts range from topical medical therapies to surgery. Many treatment modalities for anal warts are primarily focused on destroying or removing the warts locally rather than eliminating the infection [143]. There are several factors that influence the choice of treatment modality, such as location of the warts (all intra-anal or rectal warts should be managed by a specialist), number of lesions, patient's ability to apply prescribed creams or gels, patient's preference, cost of the treatment and patient's immunosuppression status.

Treatment plans can be classified either as patient self-administered modalities (for warts locat-ed on the perianal skin only) or treatment administered by a professional (for lesions in an intra-anal or rectal mucosa location).

Patient-applied treatment consists of topical medications includig podophyllin, trichloroacetic acid, bichloroacetic acid, sintecatechins and imiquimod or 5-fluorouracil that can be safely applied at home. Recurrence rates after topical medications widely range from 6.5–55%, being sinecatechins the most effective treatment with eradication rate similar to other topically applied treatments, but the lowest recurrence rate [144–146]. Moreover, patient-applied treatment side effects, which are similar for all the ointments and include redness, irritation or a burning sensation, are reported by only 1 out of 3 treated patients.

Following the center for disease control and prevention recommendations, treatments administered by a medical provider include 80–90% trichloroacetic acid (TCA) application, cryotherapy with liquid nitrogen or surgery/electrosurgery [147]. Just as for haemorrhoids, all of the procedures can be offered in an outpatient setting only to patients having small perianal warts, once the conservative treatment fails. Larger lesions require surgery performed in an operating theatre.

TCA has an erosive and chemically destructive activity; its application on AGWs burns and cauterises skin lesions. Its destructive activity may extend to nearby healthy skin, thus care must be taken during application. It is not recommended for intra-anal use. Success rates are satisfactory, ranging from 70 to 81% [148, 149], but recurrence rate is high: 36% [149].

Cryotherapy seems to be the best therapeutic. The treatment consist of freezing lesions using a liquid nitrogen cooling probe, which results in necrosis and further clearance of destroyed tissue. Complications can include the destruction of healthy skin, and ulcers or scar formation. Even if eradication and recurrence rates are similar to TCA (86% and 39% respectively) [148, 149], cryotherapy is usually preferred because it is cost effective, minimally invasive, painless and can be applied to intra-anal warts.

Surgical excision is the oldest approach, but for patients suffering from a giant condyloma (Buschke-Loewenstein tumour) it may be the treatment of choice [150, 151]. A more contemporary surgical approach, electrosurgery, is a very effective technique with a clearance rate of 94% [152] but can be painful and requires local or intravenous anaesthesia, thus cannot be performed in an ambulatory setting.

Whether specialist–applied treatment is performed in the operating room or in an ambulatory setting, it usually has satisfactory eradication rates, but also high recurrence rate, ranging from 25 to 40% [152] discouraging clinical use. Actually, all of these modalities are targeted to remove warts locally and do not destroy all the very small or subclinical lesions in the surrounding healthy-looking skin, thus increasing the risk of recurrence.

9. Skin tags

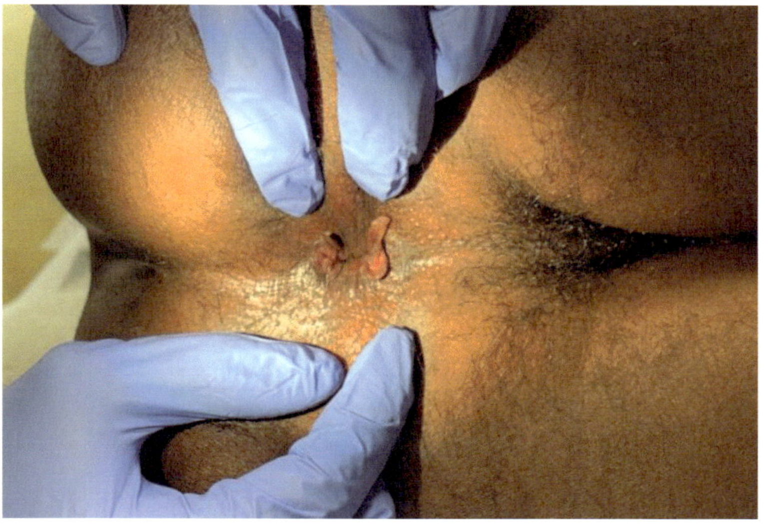

Anal skin tags are perianal skin excesses, resulting from repeated scarring, just as in case of healing from anal fissure or thrombosed external haemorrhoids, exacerbated by excess cleaning or rubbing. Affected patients are bothered by the skin excess, but usually do not complain about pain or bleeding.

Treatment includes the management of both the underlying cause and the skin lesion. The latter consists of skin tags excision easily performed as an office-based treatment, that should always follow the resolution of the underlying ano-rectal disease, to minimise the risk of recurrence.

Conflict of interest

The authors declare no conflict of interest.

Author details

Andrea Divizia[1*] and Giuseppe S. Sica[2]

1 Department of Surgical Science, Tor Vergata University, Rome, Italy

2 Gastro-Intestinal Surgery, Head Department of Surgical Science Tor Vergata University, Rome, Italy

*Address all correspondence to: andreadivizia@live.it

References

[1] Sobrado CW. Outpatient surgical proctology--past, present and future. Arq Gastroenterol. 2005;42(3):133-135. doi: 10.1590/s0004-28032005000300001

[2] Sibio S, Di Giorgio A, Campanelli M, Di Carlo S, Divizia A, Fiorani C, Scaramuzzo R, Arcudi C, Del Vecchio Blanco G, Biancone L, Sica G. Ambulatory Surgery for Perianal Crohn's Disease: Study of Feasibility. Gastroenterol Res Pract. 2018:5249087. doi: 10.1155/2018/5249087

[3] Ternent CA, Fleming F, Welton ML, Buie WD, Steele S, Rafferty J; American Society of Colon and Rectal Surgeons. Clinical Practice Guideline for Ambulatory Anorectal Surgery. Dis *Colon rectum*. 2015;58(10):915-922. doi: 10.1097/DCR.0000000000000451

[4] Gebbensleben O, Hilger Y, Rohde H. Patients' views of medical positioning for proctologic examination. Clin Exp Gastroenterol. 2009;2:133-138. doi: 10.2147/ceg.s8429

[5] Lee JH. Anesthesia for ambulatory surgery. Korean J Anesthesiol. 2017; 70(4):398-406. doi: 10.4097/kjae. 2017.70.4.398

[6] Kehlet H. Postoperative opioid sparing to hasten recovery: what are the issues? Anesthesiology. 2005;102(6):1083-1085. doi: 10.1097/00000542-200506000-00004

[7] White PF. The changing role of non-opioid analgesic techniques in the management of postoperative pain. Anesth Analg. 2005;101(5 Suppl):S5-22. doi: 10.1213/01.ane.0000177099.28914.a7

[8] Tejirian T, Abbas MA. Sitz bath: where is the evidence? Scientific basis of a common practice. Dis *Colon rectum*. 2005;48(12):2336-2340. doi: 10.1007/s10350-005-0085-x

[9] Lohsiriwat V. Treatment of hemorrhoids: A coloproctologist's view. World J Gastroenterol. 2015;21(31):9245-9252. doi: 10.3748/wjg.v21.i31.9245

[10] Jacobs D. Clinical practice. Hemorrhoids. N Engl J Med. 2014;371(10):944-951. doi: 10.1056/NEJMcp1204188

[11] van Tol RR, Kimman ML, Melenhorst J, Stassen LPS, Dirksen CD, Breukink SO; Members of the Steering Group. European Society of Coloproctology Core Outcome Set for haemorrhoidal disease: an international Delphi study among healthcare professionals. Colorectal Dis. 2019;21(5):570-580. doi: 10.1111/codi.14553

[12] van Tol RR, Kleijnen J, Watson AJM, Jongen J, Altomare DF, Qvist N, Higuero T, Muris JWM, Breukink SO. European Society of ColoProctology: guideline for haemorrhoidal disease. Colorectal Dis. 2020;22(6):650-662. doi: 10.1111/codi.14975

[13] Rho M, Guida AM, Materazzo M, Don CP, Gazia C, Ivanikhin AM, Tognoni V, Venditti D. Ligasure Hemorrhoidectomy: Updates on Complications after an 18-Year Experience. Rev Recent Clin Trials. 2020. doi: 10.2174/1574887115999201006201926

[14] Gallo G, Martellucci J, Sturiale A, Clerico G, Milito G, Marino F, Cocorullo G, Giordano P, Mistrangelo M, Trompetto M. Consensus statement of the Italian society of colorectal surgery (SICCR): management and treatment of hemorrhoidal disease. Tech Coloproctol. 2020;24(2):145-164. doi: 10.1007/s10151-020-02149-1

[15] Gallo G., Sacco R., Sammarco G. (2018) Epidemiology of Hemorrhoidal Disease. In: Ratto C., Parello A., Litta F. (eds) Hemorrhoids. Coloproctology,

2020;22(6):650-662. doi: 10.1111/codi.14975

[16] Riss S, Weiser FA, Schwameis K, Riss T, Mittlböck M, Steiner G, Stift A. The prevalence of hemorrhoids in adults. Int J Colorectal Dis. 2012; 27(2):215-220. doi: 10.1007/s00384-011-1316-3

[17] Lohsiriwat V. Hemorrhoids: from basic pathophysiology to clinical management. World J Gastroenterol. 2012;18(17):2009-17. doi: 10.3748/wjg.v18.i17.2009

[18] Trompetto M, Clerico G, Cocorullo GF, Giordano P, Marino F, Martellucci J, Milito G, Mistrangelo M, Ratto C. Evaluation and management of hemorrhoids: Italian society of colorectal surgery (SICCR) consensus statement. Tech Coloproctol. 2015;19(10):567-575. doi: 10.1007/s10151-015-1371-9

[19] Gralnek IM, Ron-Tal Fisher O, Holub JL, Eisen GM. The role of colonoscopy in evaluating hematochezia: a population-based study in a large consortium of endoscopy practices. Gastrointest Endosc. 2013;77(3):410-418. doi: 10.1016/j.gie.2012.10.025

[20] Newman J, Fitzgerald JE, Gupta S, von Roon AC, Sigurdsson HH, Allen-Mersh TG. Outcome predictors in acute surgical admissions for lower gastrointestinal bleeding. Colorectal Dis. 2012;14(8):1020-1026. doi: 10.1111/j.1463-1318.2011.02824.x

[21] Goligher JC, Leacock AG, Brossy JJ. The surgical anatomy of the anal canal. Br J Surg. 1955;43(177):51-61. doi: 10.1002/bjs.18004317707

[22] Davis BR, Lee-Kong SA, Migaly J, Feingold DL, Steele SR. The American Society of Colon and Rectal Surgeons Clinical Practice Guidelines for the Management of Hemorrhoids. Dis *Colon rectum*. 2018;61(3):284-292. doi: 10.1097/DCR.0000000000001030

[23] Marques CF, Nahas SC, Nahas CS, Sobrado CW Jr, Habr-Gama A, Kiss DR. Early results of the treatment of internal hemorrhoid disease by infrared coagulation and elastic banding: a prospective randomized cross-over trial. Tech Coloproctol. 2006;10(4):312-317. doi: 10.1007/s10151-006-0299-5

[24] Shanmugam V, Thaha MA, Rabindranath KS, Campbell KL, Steele RJ, Loudon MA. Rubber band ligation versus excisional haemorrhoidectomy for haemorrhoids. Cochrane Database Syst Rev. 2005;(3):CD005034. doi: 10.1002/14651858.CD005034

[25] Nelson RS, Ewing BM, Ternent C, Shashidharan M, Blatchford GJ, Thorson AG. Risk of late bleeding following hemorrhoidal banding in patients on antithrombotic prophylaxis. Am J Surg. 2008;196(6): 994-999; discussion 999. doi: 10.1016/j.amjsurg.2008.07.036

[26] Buchmann P, Seefeld U. Rubber band ligation for piles can be disastrous in HIV-positive patients. Int J Colorectal Dis. 1989;4(1):57-58. doi: 10.1007/BF01648552

[27] Wehrmann T, Riphaus A, Feinstein J, Stergiou N. Hemorrhoidal elastic band ligation with flexible videoendoscopes: a prospective, randomized comparison with the conventional technique that uses rigid proctoscopes. Gastrointest Endosc. 2004;60(2):191-195. doi: 10.1016/s0016-5107(04)01551-2

[28] Ramzisham AR, Sagap I, Nadeson S, Ali IM, Hasni MJ. Prospective randomized clinical trial on suction elastic band ligator versus forceps ligator in the treatment of haemorrhoids. Asian J Surg. 2005;28(4):241-245. doi: 10.1016/S1015-9584(09)60353-5

[29] Khubchandani IT. A randomized comparison of single and multiple rubber band ligations. Dis *Colon rectum*.

1983;26(11):705-708. doi: 10.1007/BF02554977

[30] Iyer VS, Shrier I, Gordon PH. Long-term outcome of rubber band ligation for symptomatic primary and recurrent internal hemorrhoids. Dis *Colon rectum*. 2004;47(8):1364-1370. doi: 10.1007/s10350-004-0591-2

[31] Beattie GC, Rao MM, Campbell WJ. Secondary haemorrhage after rubber band ligation of haemorrhoids in patients taking clopidogrel--a cautionary note. Ulster Med J. 2004;73(2):139-41. PMCID: PMC2475464

[32] Chau NG, Bhatia S, Raman M. Pylephlebitis and pyogenic liver abscesses: a complication of hemorrhoidal banding. Can J Gastroenterol. 2007;21(9):601-603. doi: 10.1155/2007/106946

[33] Tejirian T, Abbas MA. Bacterial endocarditis following rubber band ligation in a patient with a ventricular septal defect: report of a case and guideline analysis. Dis *Colon rectum*. 2006;49(12):1931-1933. doi: 10.1007/s10350-006-0769-x

[34] McCloud JM, Jameson JS, Scott AN. Life-threatening sepsis following treatment for haemorrhoids: a systematic review. Colorectal Dis. 2006;8(9):748-755. doi: 10.1111/j.1463-1318.2006.01028.x

[35] Cocorullo G, Tutino R, Falco N, Licari L, Orlando G, Fontana T, Raspanti C, Salamone G, Scerrino G, Gallo G, Trompetto M, Gulotta G. The non-surgical management for hemorrhoidal disease. A systematic review. G Chir. 2017;38(1):5-14. doi: 10.11138/gchir/2017.38.1.005

[36] Brown SR, Tiernan JP, Watson AJM, Biggs K, Shephard N, Wailoo AJ, Bradburn M, Alshreef A, Hind D; HubBLe Study team. Haemorrhoidal artery ligation versus rubber band ligation for the management of symptomatic second-degree and third-degree haemorrhoids (HubBLe): a multicentre, open-label, randomised controlled trial. Lancet. 2016;388(10042):356-364. doi: 10.1016/S0140-6736(16)30584-0

[37] Moser KH, Mosch C, Walgenbach M, Bussen DG, Kirsch J, Joos AK, Gliem P, Sauerland S. Efficacy and safety of sclerotherapy with polidocanol foam in comparison with fluid sclerosant in the treatment of first-grade haemorrhoidal disease: a randomised, controlled, single-blind, multicentre trial. Int J Colorectal Dis. 2013;28(10):1439-1447. doi: 10.1007/s00384-013-1729-2

[38] Yano T, Asano M, Tanaka S, Oda N, Matsuda Y. Prospective study comparing the new sclerotherapy and hemorrhoidectomy in terms of therapeutic outcomes at 4 years after the treatment. Surg Today. 2014;44(3):449-453. doi: 10.1007/s00595-013-0564-y

[39] Tsunoda A, Nakagi M, Kano N, Mizutani M, Yamaguchi K. Serum aluminum levels in dialysis patients after sclerotherapy of internal hemorrhoids with aluminum potassium sulfate and tannic acid. Surg Today. 2014;44(12):2314-2317. doi: 10.1007/s00595-014-0914-4

[40] Schulte T, Fändrich F, Kahlke V. Life-threatening rectal necrosis after injection sclerotherapy for haemo-rrhoids. Int J Colorectal Dis. 2008;23(7):725-726. doi: 10.1007/s00384-007-0402-z

[41] MacRae HM, McLeod RS. Compa-rison of hemorrhoidal treatments: a meta-analysis. Can J Surg. 1997;40(1):14-17. doi: 10.1007/BF02048023

[42] Gupta PJ. Infrared coagulation versus rubber band ligation in early stage hemorrhoids. Braz J Med Biol Res. 2003;36(10):1433-1439. doi: 10.1590/s0100-879x2003001000022

[43] Dimitroulopoulos D, Tsamakidis K, Xinopoulos D, Karaitianos I, Fotopoulou A, Paraskevas E. Prospective, randomized, controlled, observer-blinded trial of combined infrared photocoagulation and micronized purified flavonoid fraction versus each alone for the treatment of hemorrhoidal disease. Clin Ther. 2005;27(6):746-754. doi: 10.1016/j.clinthera.2005.06.016

[44] Lohsiriwat V. Anorectal emergencies. World J Gastroenterol. 2016;22(26):5867-5878. doi: 10.3748/wjg.v22.i26.5867

[45] Aigner F, Gruber H, Conrad F, Eder J, Wedel T, Zelger B, Engelhardt V, Lametschwandtner A, Wienert V, Böhler U, Margreiter R, Fritsch H. Revised morphology and hemo-dynamics of the anorectal vascular plexus: impact on the course of hemorrhoidal disease. Int J Colorectal Dis. 2009;24(1):105-113. doi: 10.1007/s00384-008-0572-3

[46] Grosz CR. A surgical treatment of thrombosed external hemorrhoids. Dis *Colon rectum*. 1990;33(3):249-250. doi: 10.1007/BF02134191

[47] Rivadeneira DE, Steele SR, Ternent C, Chalasani S, Buie WD, Rafferty JL; Standards Practice Task Force of The American Society of Colon and Rectal Surgeons. Practice parameters for the management of hemorrhoids (revised 2010). Dis *Colon rectum*. 2011;54(9):1059-1064. doi: 10.1097/DCR.0b013e318225513d

[48] Greenspon J, Williams SB, Young HA, Orkin BA. Thrombosed external hemorrhoids: outcome after conservative or surgical management. Dis *Colon rectum*. 2004;47(9):1493-1498. doi: 10.1007/s10350-004-0607-y.

[49] Jongen J, Bach S, Stübinger SH, Bock JU. Excision of thrombosed external hemorrhoid under local anesthesia: a retrospective evaluation of 340 patients. Dis *Colon rectum*. 2003;46(9):1226-1231. doi: 10.1007/s10350-004-6719-6

[50] PARKS AG. Pathogenesis and treatment of fistuila-in-ano. Br Med J. 1961;1(5224):463-469. doi: 10.1136/bmj.1.5224.463

[51] Gosselink MP, van Onkelen RS, Schouten WR. The cryptoglandular theory revisited. Colorectal Dis. 2015;17(12):1041-1043. doi: 10.1111/codi.13161

[52] Abcarian H. Anorectal infection: abscess-fistula. Clin Colon Rectal Surg. 2011;24(1):14-21. doi: 10.1055/s-0031-1272819

[53] Sneider EB, Maykel JA. Anal abscess and fistula. Gastroenterol Clin North Am. 2013;42(4):773-784. doi: 10.1016/j.gtc.2013.08.003

[54] Zanotti C, Martinez-Puente C, Pascual I, Pascual M, Herreros D, García-Olmo D. An assessment of the incidence of fistula-in-ano in four countries of the European Union. Int J Colorectal Dis. 2007;22(12):1459-1462. doi: 10.1007/s00384-007-0334-7

[55] Parés D. Pathogenesis and treatment of fistula in ano. Br J Surg. 2011;98(1):2-3. doi: 10.1002/bjs.7341

[56] Vogel JD, Johnson EK, Morris AM, Paquette IM, Saclarides TJ, Feingold DL, Steele SR. Clinical Practice Guideline for the Management of Anorectal Abscess, Fistula-in-Ano, and Rectovaginal Fistula. Dis *Colon rectum*. 2016;59(12):1117-1133. doi: 10.1097/DCR.0000000000000733.

[57] Amato A, Bottini C, De Nardi P, Giamundo P, Lauretta A, Realis Luc A, Tegon G, Nicholls RJ; Italian society of colorectal surgery. Evaluation and management of perianal abscess and anal fistula: a consensus statement developed by the Italian Society of Colorectal Surgery (SICCR). Tech

Coloproctol. 2015;19(10):595-606. doi: 10.1007/s10151-015-1365-7

[58] Siddiqui MR, Ashrafian H, Tozer P, Daulatzai N, Burling D, Hart A, Athanasiou T, Phillips RK. A diagnostic accuracy meta-analysis of endoanal ultrasound and MRI for perianal fistula assessment. Dis *Colon rectum*. 2012;55(5):576-585. doi: 10.1097/DCR.0b013e318249d26c

[59] Buchanan GN, Halligan S, Bartram CI, Williams AB, Tarroni D, Cohen CR. Clinical examination, endosonography, and MR imaging in preoperative assessment of fistula in ano: comparison with outcome-based reference standard. Radiology. 2004;233(3):674-681. doi: 10.1148/radiol.2333031724

[60] Pomerri F, Dodi G, Pintacuda G, Amadio L, Muzzio PC. Anal endosonography and fistulography for fistula-in-ano. Radiol Med. 2010;115(5):771-783. doi: 10.1007/s11547-010-0524-1

[61] Rizzo JA, Naig AL, Johnson EK. Anorectal abscess and fistula-in-ano: evidence-based management. Surg Clin North Am. 2010;90(1):45-68, Table of Contents. doi: 10.1016/j.suc.2009.10.001

[62] Parks AG, Gordon PH, Hardcastle JD. A classification of fistula-in-ano. Br J Surg. 1976;63(1):1-12. doi: 10.1002/bjs.1800630102

[63] Fazio VW. Complex anal fistulae. Gastroenterol Clin North Am. 1987;16(1):93-114. PMID: 3298058

[64] Schouten WR, van Vroonhoven TJ. Treatment of anorectal abscess with or without primary fistulectomy. Results of a prospective randomized trial. Dis *Colon rectum*. 1991;34(1):60-63. doi: 10.1007/BF02050209

[65] Tang CL, Chew SP, Seow-Choen F. Prospective randomized trial of drainage alone vs. drainage and fistulotomy for acute perianal abscesses with proven internal opening. Dis *Colon rectum*. 1996;39(12):1415-1417. doi: 10.1007/BF02054531

[66] Ho YH, Tan M, Chui CH, Leong A, Eu KW, Seow-Choen F. Randomized controlled trial of primary fistulotomy with drainage alone for perianal abscesses. Dis *Colon rectum*. 1997;40(12):1435-1438. doi: 10.1007/BF02070708

[67] Oliver I, Lacueva FJ, Pérez Vicente F, Arroyo A, Ferrer R, Cansado P, Candela F, Calpena R. Randomized clinical trial comparing simple drainage of anorectal abscess with and without fistula track treatment. Int J Colorectal Dis. 2003;18(2):107-110. doi: 10.1007/s00384-002-0429-0

[68] Malik AI, Nelson RL, Tou S. Incision and drainage of perianal abscess with or without treatment of anal fistula. Cochrane Database Syst Rev. 2010;(7):CD006827. doi: 10.1002/14651858.CD006827.pub2

[69] Sawyer RG, Claridge JA, Nathens AB, Rotstein OD, Duane TM, Evans HL, Cook CH, O'Neill PJ, Mazuski JE, Askari R, Wilson MA, Napolitano LM, Namias N, Miller PR, Dellinger EP, Watson CM, Coimbra R, Dent DL, Lowry SF, Cocanour CS, West MA, Banton KL, Cheadle WG, Lipsett PA, Guidry CA, Popovsky K; STOP-IT Trial Investigators. Trial of short-course antimicrobial therapy for intraabdominal infection. N Engl J Med. 2015;372(21):1996-2005. doi: 10.1056/NEJMoa1411162

[70] Mocanu V, Dang JT, Ladak F, Tian C, Wang H, Birch DW, Karmali S. Antibiotic use in prevention of anal fistulas following incision and drainage of anorectal abscesses: A systematic review and meta-analysis. Am J Surg. 2019;217(5):910-917. doi: 10.1016/j.amjsurg.2019.01.015

[71] de Groof EJ, Cabral VN, Buskens CJ, Morton DG, Hahnloser D, Bemelman WA; research committee of the European Society of Coloproctology. Systematic review of evidence and consensus on perianal fistula: an analysis of national and international guidelines. Colorectal Dis. 2016;18(4):O119–O134. doi: 10.1111/codi.13286

[72] Hammond TM, Knowles CH, Porrett T, Lunniss PJ. The Snug Seton: short and medium term results of slow fistulotomy for idiopathic anal fistulae. Colorectal Dis. 2006;8(4):328-337. doi: 10.1111/j.1463-1318.2005.00926.x

[73] Dziki A, Bartos M. Seton treatment of anal fistula: experience with a new modification. Eur J Surg. 1998;164(7):543-548. doi: 10.1080/110241598750005930

[74] Quah HM, Tang CL, Eu KW, Chan SY, Samuel M. Meta-analysis of randomized clinical trials comparing drainage alone vs primary sphincter-cutting procedures for anorectal abscess-fistula. Int J Colorectal Dis. 2006;21(6):602-609. doi: 10.1007/s00384-005-0060-y

[75] Hall JF, Bordeianou L, Hyman N, Read T, Bartus C, Schoetz D, Marcello PW. Outcomes after operations for anal fistula: results of a prospective, multicenter, regional study. Dis *Colon rectum*. 2014;57(11):1304-1308. doi: 10.1097/DCR.0000000000000216

[76] Abramowitz L, Soudan D, Souffran M, Bouchard D, Castinel A, Suduca JM, Staumont G, Devulder F, Pigot F, Ganansia R, Varastet M; Groupe de Recherche en Proctologie de la Société Nationale Française de Colo-Proctologie and the Club de Réflexion des Cabinets et Groupe d'Hépato-Gastroentérologie. The outcome of fistulotomy for anal fistula at 1 year: a prospective multicentre French study. Colorectal Dis. 2016;18(3):279-285. doi: 10.1111/codi.13121

[77] Davies M, Harris D, Lohana P, Chandra Sekaran TV, Morgan AR, Beynon J, Carr ND. The surgical management of fistula-in-ano in a specialist colorectal unit. Int J Colorectal Dis. 2008;23(9):833-838. doi: 10.1007/s00384-008-0444-x

[78] Westerterp M, Volkers NA, Poolman RW, van Tets WF. Anal fistulotomy between Skylla and Charybdis. Colorectal Dis. 2003;5(6): 549-551. doi: 10.1046/j.1463-1318.2003.00459.x

[79] Ho KS, Tsang C, Seow-Choen F, Ho YH, Tang CL, Heah SM, Eu KW. Prospective randomised trial comparing ayurvedic cutting seton and fistulotomy for low fistula-in-ano. Tech Coloproctol. 2001;5(3):137-141. doi: 10.1007/s101510100015

[80] Christensen A, Nilas L, Christiansen J. Treatment of trans-sphincteric anal fistulas by the seton technique. Dis *Colon rectum*. 1986; 29(7):454-455. doi: 10.1007/BF02561583

[81] van Koperen PJ, Wind J, Bemelman WA, Bakx R, Reitsma JB, Slors JF. Long-term functional outcome and risk factors for recurrence after surgical treatment for low and high perianal fistulas of cryptoglandular origin. Dis *Colon rectum*. 2008;51(10): 1475-1481. doi: 10.1007/s10350-008-9354-9

[82] Jordán J, Roig JV, García-Armengol J, García-Granero E, Solana A, Lledó S. Risk factors for recurrence and incontinence after anal fistula surgery. Colorectal Dis. 2010;12(3):254-260. doi: 10.1111/j.1463-1318.2009.01806.x

[83] Kelly ME, Heneghan HM, McDermott FD, Nason GJ, Freeman C, Martin ST, Winter DC. The role of loose seton in the management of anal fistula: a multicenter study of 200 patients. Tech Coloproctol. 2014;18(10):915-919. doi: 10.1007/s10151-014-1186-0

[84] Williams JG, MacLeod CA, Rothenberger DA, Goldberg SM. Seton treatment of high anal fistulae. Br J Surg. 1991;78(10):1159-1161. doi: 10.1002/bjs.1800781004

[85] Patton V, Chen CM, Lubowski D. Long-term results of the cutting seton for high anal fistula. ANZ J Surg. 2015;85(10):720-727. doi: 10.1111/ans.13156

[86] Rosen DR, Kaiser AM. Definitive seton management for transsphincteric fistula-in-ano: harm or charm? Colorectal Dis. 2016;18(5):488-495. doi: 10.1111/codi.13120

[87] Ritchie RD, Sackier JM, Hodde JP. Incontinence rates after cutting seton treatment for anal fistula. Colorectal Dis. 2009;11(6):564-571. doi: 10.1111/j.1463-1318.2008.01713.x

[88] Rojanasakul A, Pattanaarun J, Sahakitrungruang C, Tantiphlachiva K. Total anal sphincter saving technique for fistula-in-ano; the ligation of intersphincteric fistula tract. J Med Assoc Thai. 2007;90(3):581-586

[89] Shanwani A, Nor AM, Amri N. Ligation of the intersphincteric fistula tract (LIFT): a sphincter-saving technique for fistula-in-ano. Dis *Colon rectum*. 2010;53(1):39-42. doi: 10.1007/DCR.0b013e3181c160c4

[90] Yellinek S, Krizzuk D, Moreno Djadou T, Lavy D, Wexner SD. Endorectal advancement flap for complex anal fistula: does flap configuration matter? Colorectal Dis. 2019;21(5):581-587. doi: 10.1111/codi.14564

[91] Podetta M, Scarpa CR, Zufferey G, Skala K, Ris F, Roche B, Buchs NC. Mucosal advancement flap for recurrent complex anal fistula: a repeatable procedure. Int J Colorectal Dis. 2019;34(1):197-200. doi: 10.1007/s00384-018-3155-y

[92] Lightner AL, Vogel JD, Carmichael JC, Keller DS, Shah SA, Mahadevan U, Kane SV, Paquette IM, Steele SR, Feingold DL. The American Society of Colon and Rectal Surgeons Clinical Practice Guidelines for the Surgical Management of Crohn's Disease. Dis *Colon rectum*. 2020;63(8):1028-1052. doi: 10.1097/DCR.0000000000001716

[93] Strong SA, Koltun WA, Hyman NH, Buie WD; Standards Practice Task Force of The American Society of Colon and Rectal Surgeons. Practice parameters for the surgical management of Crohn's disease. Dis *Colon rectum*. 2007;50(11):1735-1746. doi: 10.1007/s10350-007-9012-7

[94] Strong S, Steele SR, Boutrous M, Bordineau L, Chun J, Stewart DB, Vogel J, Rafferty JF; Clinical Practice Guidelines Committee of the American Society of Colon and Rectal Surgeons. Clinical Practice Guideline for the Surgical Management of Crohn's Disease. Dis *Colon rectum*. 2015;58(11):1021-1036. doi: 10.1097/DCR.0000000000000450

[95] Petagna L, Antonelli A, Ganini C, Bellato V, Campanelli M, Divizia A, Efrati C, Franceschilli M, Guida AM, Ingallinella S, Montagnese F, Sensi B, Siragusa L, Sica GS. Pathophysiology of Crohn's disease inflammation and recurrence. Biol Direct. 2020;15(1):23. doi: 10.1186/s13062-020-00280-5.

[96] Schwartz DA, Loftus EV Jr, TremaineWJ,PanaccioneR,HarmsenWS, Zinsmeister AR, Sandborn WJ. The natural history of fistulizing Crohn's disease in Olmsted County, Minnesota. Gastroenterology. 2002;122(4):875-880. doi: 10.1053/gast.2002.32362

[97] Sica GS, Di Carlo S, Tema G, Montagnese F, Del Vecchio Blanco G, Fiaschetti V, Maggi G, Biancone L. Treatment of peri-anal fistula in Crohn's disease. World J Gastroenterol.

2014;20(37):13205-13210. doi: 10.3748/wjg.v20.i37.13205

[98] Singh B, McC Mortensen NJ, Jewell DP, George B. Perianal Crohn's disease. Br J Surg. 2004;91(7):801-814. doi: 10.1002/bjs.4613

[99] van der Hagen SJ, Baeten CG, Soeters PB, van Gemert WG. Long-term outcome following mucosal advancement flap for high perianal fistulas and fistulotomy for low perianal fistulas: recurrent perianal fistulas: failure of treatment or recurrent patient disease? Int J Colorectal Dis. 2006;21(8):784-790. doi: 10.1007/s00384-005-0072-7

[100] A. M. Scanu, Fistole perianali nella malattia di Crohn iter formativo in coloproctologia corso avanzato e update in colo proctologia. [Internet] Vercelli, 2008. Available from: https://www.siccr.org/wp-content/uploads/2015/08/scanu_doc.pdf [Accessed: 2008-12-15/17]

[101] Ingallinella S, Campanelli M, Antonelli A, Arcudi C, Bellato V, Divizia A, Franceschilli M, Petagna L, Sensi B, Sibio S, Siragusa L, Sica GS. The Role of Active Inflammation and Surgical Therapy in Crohn's Disease Recurrence. Gastroenterol Res Pract. 2020;2020:2845407. doi: 10.1155/2020/2845407

[102] L. Biancone, S. Onali, E. Calabrese, C. Petruzziello, F. Zorzi, G. Condino, G.S. Sica, F. Pallone. Non-invasive techniques for assessing postoperative recurrence in Crohn's disease. Dig Liver Dis. 2008;40,(2):265-270. doi: 10.1016/S1590-8658(08)60536-8

[103] Lee MJ, Freer C, Adegbola S, Elkady S, Parkes M, Hart A, Fearnhead NS, Lobo AJ, Brown SR. Patients with perianal Crohn's fistulas experience delays in accessing anti-TNF therapy due to slow recognition, diagnosis and integration of specialist services: lessons learned from three referral centres. Colorectal Dis. 2018;20(9):797-803. doi: 10.1111/codi.14102

[104] Gold SL, Cohen-Mekelburg S, Schneider Y, Steinlauf A. Perianal Fistulas in Patients With Crohn's Disease, Part 1: Current Medical Management. Gastroenterol Hepatol (N Y). 2018;14(8):470-481. PMID: 30302062

[105] Sica GS, Biancone L. Surgery for inflammatory bowel disease in the era of laparoscopy. World J Gastroenterol. 2013;19(16):2445-2448. doi: 10.3748/wjg.v19.i16.2445

[106] Comparative study of laparoscopic vs open gastrectomy in gastric cancer management Sica, G.S., Iaculli, E., Biancone, L., di Carlo, S., Scaramuzzo, R., Fiorani, C., Gentileschi, P., Gaspari, A.L. World Journal of Gastroenterology. 2011;17(41):4602-4606. doi: 10.3748/wjg.v17.i41.4602

[107] EuroSurg Collaborative. EuroSurg: a new European student-driven research network in surgery. Colorectal Dis. 2016 Feb;18(2):214-215. doi:10.1111/codi.13260

[108] D'Ugo S, Romano F, Sibio S, Bagaglini G, Sensi B, Biancone L, Monteleone G, Sica GS. Impact of surgery on quality of life in Crohn's disease: short- and mid-term follow-up. Updates Surg. 2020;72(3):773-780. doi: 10.1007/s13304-020-00738-1

[109] Divizia A, Sensi B, Sica GS. Ambulatory management of perianal Crohn's disease during the COVID-19 pandemic. Colorectal Dis. 2020;22(6):645-646. doi: 10.1111/codi.15104

[110] Torres J, Bonovas S, Doherty G, Kucharzik T, Gisbert JP, Raine T, Adamina M, Armuzzi A, Bachmann O, Bager P, Biancone L, BokemeyerB,BossuytP,BurischJ,CollinsP, El-Hussuna A, Ellul P, Frei-Lanter C, Furfaro F, Gingert C, Gionchetti P,

Gomollon F, González-Lorenzo M, Gordon H, Hlavaty T, Juillerat P, Katsanos K, Kopylov U, Krustins E, Lytras T, Maaser C, Magro F, Marshall JK, Myrelid P, Pellino G, Rosa I, Sabino J, Savarino E, Spinelli A, Stassen L, Uzzan M, Vavricka S, Verstockt B, Warusavitarne J, Zmora O, Fiorino G. ECCO Guidelines on Therapeutics in Crohn's Disease: Medical Treatment. J Crohns Colitis. 2020;14(1):4-22. doi: 10.1093/ecco-jcc/jjz180

[111] Franzè E, Monteleone I, Laudisi F, Rizzo A, Dinallo V, Di Fusco D, Colantoni A, Ortenzi A, Giuffrida P, Di Carlo S, Sica GS, Di Sabatino A, Monteleone G. Cadherin-11 Is a Regulator of Intestinal Fibrosis. J Crohns Colitis. 2020;14(3):406-417. doi: 10.1093/ecco-jcc/jjz147

[112] Franzè E, Dinallo V, Laudisi F, Di Grazia A, Di Fusco D, Colantoni A, Ortenzi A, Giuffrida P, Di Carlo S, Sica GS, Di Sabatino A, Monteleone G. Interleukin-34 Stimulates Gut Fibroblasts to Produce Collagen Synthesis. J Crohns Colitis. 2020;14(10):1436-1445. doi: 10.1093/ecco-jcc/jjaa073

[113] Franzè E, Di Grazia A, Sica GS, Biancone L, Laudisi F, Monteleone G. Interleukin-34 Enhances the Tumor Promoting Function of Colorectal Cancer-Associated Fibroblasts. Cancers (Basel). 2020;12(12):3537. doi: 10.3390/cancers12123537

[114] Franzè, E., Dinallo, V., Rizzo, A., Di Giovangiulio, M., Bevivino, G., Stolfi, C., Caprioli, F., Colantoni, A., Ortenzi, A., Di Grazia, A., Sica, G., Sileri, P., Rossi, P., Monteleone, G. Interleukin-34 sustains pro-tumorigenic signals in colon cancer tissue. Oncotarget. 2018;9(3):3432-3445

[115] Interleukin-34 Induces Cc-chemokine Ligand 20 in Gut Epithelial Cells. Franzè E, Marafini I, De Simone V, Monteleone I, Caprioli F, Colantoni A,Ortenzi A, Crescenzi F, Izzo R, Sica G, Sileri P, Rossi P, Pallone F, MonteleoneG.J.CrohnsColitis.2016;10(1):87-94. doi: 10.1093/ecco-jcc/jjv181

[116] Interleukin-25 production is differently regulated by TNF-alpha and TGF-beta 1 in the human gut. Fina D, Franze E, Rovedatti L, Corazza GR, Biancone L, Sileri PP, Sica G, MacDonald TT, Pallone F, Di Sabatino A, Monteleone G. Mucosal Immunology, 2011;4(2):239-44 doi: 10.1038/mi.2010.68

[117] Haggett PJ, Moore NR, Shearman JD, Travis SP, Jewell DP, Mortensen NJ. Pelvic and perineal complications of Crohn's disease: assessment using magnetic resonance imaging. Gut. 1995;36(3):407-410. doi: 10.1136/gut.36.3.407

[118] Buchanan GN, Halligan S, Bartram CI, Williams AB, Tarroni D, Cohen CR. Clinical examination, endosonography, and MR imaging in preoperative assessment of fistula in ano: comparison with outcome-based reference standard. Radiology. 2004;233(3):674-681. doi: 10.1148/radiol.2333031724

[119] Sloots CE, Felt-Bersma RJ, Poen AC, Cuesta MA, Meuwissen SG. Assessment and classification of fistula-in-ano in patients with Crohn's disease by hydrogen peroxide enhanced transanal ultrasound. Int J Colorectal Dis. 2001;16(5):292-297. doi: 10.1007/s003840100308

[120] Lee MJ, Heywood N, Sagar PM, Brown SR, Fearnhead NS; ACPGBI Perianal Crohn's Disease Group. Association of Coloproctology of Great Britain and Ireland consensus exercise on surgical management of fistulating perianal Crohn's disease. Colorectal Dis. 2017;19(5):418-429. doi: 10.1111/codi.13672

[121] Onali S, Calabrese E, Petruzziello C, Zorzi F, Sica GS, Lolli E, Ascolani M, Condino G, Pallone F, Biancone L. Endoscopic vs ultrasonographic findings related to Crohn's disease recurrence: a

prospective longitudinal study at 3 years. J Crohns Colitis. 2010;4(3):319-328. doi: 10.1016/j.crohns.2009.12.010

[122] Al-Khawari HA, Gupta R, Sinan TS, Prakash B, Al-Amer A, Al-Bolushi S. Role of magnetic resonance imaging in the assessment of perianal fistulas. Med Princ Pract. 2005;14(1):46-52. doi: 10.1159/000081923

[123] Sandborn WJ, Fazio VW, Feagan BG, Hanauer SB; American Gastroenterological Association Clinical Practice Committee. AGA technical review on perianal Crohn's disease. Gastroenterology. 2003;125(5):1508-1530. doi: 10.1016/j.gastro.2003.08.025

[124] Gecse KB, Bemelman W, Kamm MA, Stoker J, Khanna R, Ng SC, Panés J, van Assche G, Liu Z, Hart A, Levesque BG, D'Haens G; World Gastroenterology Organization, International Organisation for Inflammatory Bowel Diseases IOIBD, European Society of Coloproctology and Robarts Clinical Trials; World Gastroenterology Organization International Organisation for Inflammatory Bowel Diseases IOIBD European Society of Coloproctology and Robarts Clinical Trials. A global consensus on the classification, diagnosis and multidisciplinary treatment of perianal fistulising Crohn's disease. Gut. 2014;63(9):1381-92. doi: 10.1136/gutjnl-2013-306709

[125] Kotze PG, Shen B, Lightner A, Yamamoto T, Spinelli A, Ghosh S, Panaccione R. Modern management of perianal fistulas in Crohn's disease: future directions. Gut. 2018;67(6):1181-1194. doi: 10.1136/gutjnl-2017-314918

[126] Pellino G, Keller DS, Sampietro GM, Angriman I, Carvello M, Celentano V, Colombo F, Di Candido F, Laureti S, Luglio G, Poggioli G, Rottoli M, Scaringi S, Sciaudone G, Sica G, Sofo L, Leone S, Danese S, Spinelli A, Delaini G, Selvaggi F; Italian Society of Colorectal Surgery SICCR. Inflammatory bowel disease position statement of the Italian Society of Colorectal Surgery (SICCR): Crohn's disease. Tech Coloproctol. 2020;24(5):421-448. doi: 10.1007/s10151-020-02183-z

[127] Pellino G, Selvaggi F, Ghezzi G, Corona D, Riegler G, Delaini GG. A think tank of the Italian society of colorectal surgery (SICCR) on the surgical treatment of inflammatory bowel disease using the Delphi method: Crohn's disease. Tech Coloproctol. 2015;19(10):639-651. doi: 10.1007/s10151-015-1368-4

[128] Adamina M, Bonovas S, Raine T, Spinelli A, Warusavitarne J, Armuzzi A, Bachmann O, Bager P, Biancone L, Bokemeyer B, Bossuyt P, Burisch J, Collins P, Doherty G, El-Hussuna A, Ellul P, Fiorino G, Frei-Lanter C, Furfaro F, Gingert C, Gionchetti P, Gisbert JP, Gomollon F, González Lorenzo M, Gordon H, Hlavaty T, Juillerat P, Katsanos K, Kopylov U, Krustins E, Kucharzik T, Lytras T, Maaser C, Magro F, Marshall JK, Myrelid P, Pellino G, Rosa I, Sabino J, Savarino E, Stassen L, Torres J, Uzzan M, Vavricka S, Verstockt B, Zmora O. ECCO Guidelines on Therapeutics in Crohn's Disease: Surgical Treatment. J Crohns Colitis. 2020;14(2):155-168. doi: 10.1093/ecco-jcc/jjz187

[129] Ommer A, Herold A, Berg E, Fürst A, Post S, Ruppert R, Schiedeck T, Schwandner O, Strittmatter B. German S3 guidelines: anal abscess and fistula (second revised version). Langenbecks Arch Surg. 2017;402(2):191-201. doi: 10.1007/s00423-017-1563-z

[130] Koelbel G, Schmiedl U, Majer MC, Weber P, Jenss H, Kueper K, Hess CF. Diagnosis of fistulae and sinus tracts in patients with Crohn disease: value of MR imaging. AJR Am J Roentgenol. 1989;152(5):999-1003. doi: 10.2214/ajr.152.5.999

[131] Bouchard D, Abramowitz L, Bouguen G, Brochard C, Dabadie A,

de Parades V, Eléouet-Kaplan M, Fathallah N, Faucheron JL, Maggiori L, Panis Y, Pigot F, Rouméguère P, Sénéjoux A, Siproudhis L, Staumont G, Suduca JM, Vinson-Bonnet B, Zeitoun JD. Anoperineal lesions in Crohn's disease: French recommendations for clinical practice. Tech Coloproctol. 2017;21(9):683-691. doi: 10.1007/s10151-017-1684-y

[132] Orsoni P, Barthet M, Portier F, Panuel M, Desjeux A, Grimaud JC. Prospective comparison of endosonography, magnetic resonance imaging and surgical findings in anorectal fistula and abscess complicating Crohn's disease. Br J Surg. 1999;86(3):360-364. doi: 10.1046/j.1365-2168.1999.01020.x

[133] Bemelman WA, Warusavitarne J, Sampietro GM, Serclova Z, Zmora O, Luglio G, de Buck van Overstraeten A, Burke JP, Buskens CJ, Colombo F, Dias JA, Eliakim R, Elosua T, Gecim IE, Kolacek S, Kierkus J, Kolho KL, Lefevre JH, Millan M, Panis Y, Pinkney T, Russell RK, Shwaartz C, Vaizey C, Yassin N, D'Hoore A. ECCO-ESCP Consensus on Surgery for Crohn's Disease. J Crohns Colitis. 2018;12(1):1-16. doi: 10.1093/ecco-jcc/jjx061

[134] Sibio S, Di Giorgio A, Campanelli M, Di Carlo S, Divizia A, Fiorani C, Scaramuzzo R, Arcudi C, Del Vecchio Blanco G, Biancone L, Sica G. Ambulatory Surgery for Perianal Crohn's Disease: Study of Feasibility. Gastroenterol Res Pract. 2018;5249087. doi: 10.1155/2018/5249087

[135] An Y, Bellato V, Konishi T, Pellino G, Sensi B, Siragusa L, Franceschilli M, Sica GS; S-COVID Collaborative Group. Surgeons' fear of getting infected by COVID19: A global survey. Br J Surg. 2020;107(11):e543-e544. doi: 10.1002/bjs.11833

[136] Bellato V, Konishi T, Pellino G, An Y, Piciocchi A, Sensi B, Siragusa L, Khanna K, Pirozzi BM, Franceschilli M, Campanelli M, Efetov S, Sica GS; S-COVID Collaborative Group. Impact of asymptomatic COVID-19 patients in global surgical practice during the COVID-19 pandemic. Br J Surg. 2020;107(10):e364-e365. doi: 10.1002/bjs.11800

[137] Sensi B, Siragusa L, Efrati C, Petagna L, Franceschilli M, Bellato V, Antonelli A, Arcudi C, Campanelli M, Ingallinella S, Guida AM, Divizia A. The Role of Inflammation in Crohn's Disease Recurrence after Surgical Treatment. J Immunol Res. 2020;2020:8846982. doi: 10.1155/2020/8846982

[138] Sileri P, Sica G, Gentileschi P, Venza M, Manzelli A, Palmieri G, Spagnoli LG, Testa G, Benedetti E, Gaspari AL. Ischemic preconditioning protects intestine from prolonged ischemia. Transplant Proc. 2004;36(2):283-285. doi: 10.1016/j.transproceed.2004.01.078

[139] Sica, G.S., Djapardy, V., Westaby, S., Maynard, N.D. Diagnosis and management of aortoesophageal fistula caused by a foreign body. Annals of Thoracic Surgery. 2004;77(6):2217-2218 doi: 10.1016/j.athoracsur.2003.06.031

[140] Baseman JG, Koutsky LA. The epidemiology of human papillomavirus infections. J Clin Virol. 2005;32 Suppl 1:S16–S24. doi: 10.1016/j.jcv.2004.12.008

[141] Kreisel KM, Spicknall IH, Gargano JW, Lewis FM, Lewis RM, Markowitz LE, Roberts H, Satcher Johnson A, Song R, St Cyr SB, Weston EJ, Torrone EA, Weinstock HS. Sexually Transmitted Infections Among US Women and Men: Prevalence and Incidence Estimates, 2018. Sex Transm Dis. 2021. doi: 10.1097/OLQ.0000000000001355.

[142] Sturegard E, Johansson H, Ekstrom J, Hasson BG, Johnsson A, Gustafsson E, Dillner J, Forslund O.

Human papillomavirus typing in reporting condyloma. Sex Transm dis 2013;40:123-129. doi: 10.1097/OLQ.0b013e31827aa9b3.

[143] Lee PK, Bas Wilkins K. Condyloma and other infections including human immunodeficiency virus. Surg clin N am 2010;90:99-112. doi: 10.1016/j.suc.2009.09.005.

[144] Lacey CJN, Goodall RL, Rangarson Tennvall G, Maw R, Kinghorn GR, Fisk PG, Barton S, Byren I. Randomised controlled trial and economic evaluation of podophyllotoxin solution, podophyllotoxin cream, and podophyllin in the treatment of genital warts. Sex Transm Infect 2003;79:270-275. doi: 10.1136/sti.79.4.270.

[145] Edwards A, Atma-Ram A, Thin RN. Podophyllotoxin 0.5% v. podophyllin 20% to treat penile warts. Genitourin Med 1988;64:263-265. doi: 10.1136/sti.64.4.263.

[146] Tatti S, Stockfleth E, Beutner KR, Tawfik K, Elsasser U, Weyrauch P, Mescheder A. Polyphenon E: a new treat-ment for external anogenital warts. Br J dermatol 2010;162:176-184.

[147] STd Treatment Guidelines [Internet]. Available from: www.cdc.gov/std/treatment/2010/genital-warts.htm

[148] Abdullah AN, Walzman M, Wade A. Treatment of external genital warts comparing cryotherapy (liquid nitro-gen) and trichloroacetic acid. Sex Transm dis 1993;20:344-345. PMID: 8108758

[149] Godley MJ, Bradbeer CS, Gellan M, Thin RN. Cryotherapy compared with tricholoroacetic acid in treating geni-tal warts. Genitourin Med 1987;63:390-392. doi: 10.1136/sti.63.6.390.

[150] Balik E, Eren T, Bugra D. A surgical approach to anogenital buschke-Loewenstein tumours (giant condyloma acuminate). Acta chir belgica 2009;109:612-616. doi: 10.1080/00015458.2009.11680497.

[151] Paraskevas KI, Kyriakos E, Poulios V, Stathopoulos A, Tzovaras A, Briana DD. Surgical management of giant condyloma acuminatum (Suschke-Loewenstein tumor) of the perianal region. Dermatol Surg 2007;33:638-644. doi: 10.1111/j.1524-4725.2007.33125.x.

[152] Stone KM, Becker TM, Hadgu A, Kraus SJ. Treatment of external genital warts: a randomised clinical trial comparing podophyllin, cryotherapy, and electrodesiccation. Genitourin Med. 1990;66(1):16-19. doi: 10.1136/sti.66.1.16.